T0144743

GREENS
ARE GOOD
FOR YOU!

HOW GREEN POWER PROTECTS YOU AGAINST:
- *Heart Disease* • *Cancer*
- *Diabetes* • *Macular Degeneration*
- *Poor Night Vision* • *Senile Dementia*
- *Liver Disease* • *Fatigue*
- *Blood, Sleep, Urinary, and Colorectal Disorders*

Earl L. Mindell, R.Ph., Ph.D.
& Tony O'Donnell

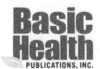

Basic Health
PUBLICATIONS, INC.

The information contained in this book is based upon the research and personal and professional experiences of the authors. It is not intended as a substitute for consulting with your physician or other healthcare provider. Any attempt to diagnose and treat an illness should be done under the direction of a healthcare professional.

The publisher does not advocate the use of any particular healthcare protocol but believes the information in this book should be available to the public. The publisher and authors are not responsible for any adverse effects or consequences resulting from the use of the suggestions, preparations, or procedures discussed in this book. Should the reader have any questions concerning the appropriateness of any procedures or preparation mentioned, the authors and the publisher strongly suggest consulting a professional healthcare advisor.

Series Cover Designer: Mike Stromberg
Editor: Linda Comac
Typesetter: Gary A. Rosenberg

Basic Health Guides are published by
Basic Health Publications, Inc.

Printed in the USA
CPSIA information can be obtained
at www.ICGtesting.com
JSHW012009140824
68134JS00004B/100

CONTENTS

INTRODUCTION

Inevitably, eyesight diminishes with advancing age. The incidence of eye disease jumps by ten times among older people. Couple this with the fact that we are living longer, into our seventh and eighth decades of life, and it doesn't take long to understand that the challenge of treating eye disease now and in the future is going to be very burdensome.

The focusing lens of the eye loses 1 percent of its transparency for every year of life until, by age sixty, about two-thirds of us show signs of early cataracts. By age eighty, an adult will need a 200-watt light bulb to visualize reading materials compared to when they were twenty years old and only needed a sixty-watt bulb to read indoors. For most Americans, a cataract operation is in their future.

Cataracts
An opacity or cloudiness in the normally clear crystalline lens used for focusing on near objects.

Glaucoma is a "sneak thief of sight" because it slowly robs a person of their side vision without becoming apparent to most adults. Half the cases go undetected. Although current treatments, such as eye drops and laser treatments, may reduce abnormally high fluid pressure that could destroy the optic nerve, in the long run, many adults still develop this severe visual disability. While only about 2 percent of adults over age forty have glaucoma, this figure jumps up to more than 5 to

12 percent in the older age brackets. And even the best treatment does not address the form of glaucoma caused by nerve toxins.

Diabetes affects about 8 to 12 percent of American adults. The rate of diabetes is rising so fast in the United States that it has health authorities alarmed, if for no other reason than that severe visual problems are highly prevalent among adults who have trouble regulating blood sugar. Swelling and hemorrhaging at the back of the eyes, along with sugar cataracts, often cause severe visual handicaps in people with diabetes.

Macular degeneration is still one of the most depressing eye disorders because often people don't discover it until they close one eye and discover that their other eye can no longer see objects in its central visual field. Then their eye doctor makes the diagnosis of macular degeneration and indicates there is nothing that can be done to restore the lost vision. Worse yet, in a four-year period of time, the problem may spread to the opposing eye. About a third of older Americans exhibit early signs of macular disease and about 9 percent have actually lost central vision.

The most common eye problem seen in eye doctors' offices is dry eye. Doctors tend to dismiss it as a trivial problem, but it is the most irritating because dry eyes make it impossible to wear contact lenses, and artificial tear preparations provide only temporary relief.

The good news is that there are natural therapies for all these eye disorders that are often overlooked by conventional medicine. Given that the loss of sight is the number two health fear behind cancer, it would behoove all Americans to learn more about preventive eye care.

It's never too late to begin learning about healthy foods and food supplements for the eyes. Even if you have lost some vision, nutritional therapy may help you hang on to your remaining vision.

Nutrition can be so confusing to understand. There are plenty of research studies, but can we plan a course of action from these studies? Do we just eat more plant foods, or do we need food supplements to reduce our risk of age-related vision loss?

There are many newly published reports on how nutritional factors may be beneficial for your eyes, and it's now time to put into practice what we know about nutrition and the eyes. This book will help you to do that.

Most of the nutritional research regarding eye health is centered on antioxidants, the anti-rusting agents. These antioxidants work in tandem, that is, they work better together rather than alone. For example, vitamin E donates an electron to prevent fatty tissues in the eyes from becoming oxidized, but in doing so it becomes oxidized itself. So, along comes vitamin C, which donates an electron to vitamin E and reactivates it. And, bioflavonoid pigments, such as bilberry, blueberry, and cranberry, help to maintain vitamin C levels in the eyes, so they are synergistic. The trace mineral selenium combines with vitamin E to produce an antioxidant enzyme (glutathione peroxidase) that cleans up cellular debris at the back of the eyes. Along with vitamin C, glutathione and lutein are probably the most potent nutritional remedies for eye disease today, but there are many others, so you don't need to become fixated on any single nutrient.

It helps to know the nutritional geography of the eyes. Which nutrients are found in the various eye structures and how are they involved in preventing eye disorders? Here is a brief overview of the tissues of the eyes and the potentially beneficial nutrients for them.

- Aqueous fluid: glutathione, lutein, vitamin C, vitamin E

- Blood supply (choroid and blood capillaries): bilberry, ginkgo biloba, magnesium

- Bruch's membrane: mineral chelators, such as IP_6 rice-bran extract

- Cornea: coenzyme Q_{10}, collagen, hyaluronic acid

- Fluid drain of the eyes (trabecular meshwork): hyaluronic acid, vitamin C

- Focusing lens (where cataracts occur): glutathione, lutein, vitamin C, vitamin E

- Optic nerve: glutathione, vitamin B_{12}

- Photoreceptor cells (where macular degeneration and night blindness occur): DHA/omega-3 oils, rods and cones, vitamin A

- Retinal cleansing cells (retinal pigment epithelium): selenium and vitamin E

- Retinal nerve layer: glutathione, hyaluronic acid, lutein, and zeaxanthin

- Sclera (white of the eyes): collagen, hyaluronic acid, iron, proline, vitamin C

- Tear film: essential oils for oily layer, vitamin A for mucin

- Vitreous jelly (where floaters occur): hyaluronic acid, water

People frequently ask, can't I just eat the right foods and keep my vision? Yes, foods are very important for the maintenance of sight. For example, there is a plant-pigment duo, lutein and its cousin zeaxanthin, which is lacking in many diets unless a person consumes a lot of spinach or kale. And with advancing age, the eyes need more antioxidant protection from lutein and zeaxanthin than can be provided by foods alone. Food supplements do not replace a good diet, nor does the best plant food diet eliminate the need for vitamin supplements. Some people simply don't like swallowing vitamin pills, even though they are less problematic and less expensive than many prescription medications. The sooner you begin a food and food-supplement regimen to help maintain your vision, the better off you will be.

CHAPTER 1

VITAMINS

Vitamins are essential nutritional factors for health. They are grouped into watery (dissolve in water) and fatty (dissolve in fat) vitamins. The water-soluble vitamins include vitamin C and the array of B vitamins. The fat-soluble vitamins are vitamins A, D, E, and K, which are stored in tissues and liver for later use.

Vitamins
Organic substances occurring in small amounts in foods that are required for health.

Vitamin A

Vitamin A plays an essential role in ocular health, both at the front and back of the eyes. Supplemental vitamin A can be both beneficial and potentially troublesome.

Vitamin A for the Front of the Eyes

Vitamin A is required for the production of mucin from glands in the eyelids. Mucin helps the tear film to spread across the cornea and keep it moist. Low mucin levels can result in filmy strands of material inside the eyelids.

Low vitamin A intake may result in foamy gray triangular spots on the conjunctiva, the clear film that covers the surface of the eyes just beneath the eyelids. These are called Bitot's spots and are seen primarily in cases of malnutrition. A severe deficiency of vitamin A results in a condition called xerophthalmia, which produces symptoms of corneal dryness and ulceration.

Vitamin A for the Back of the Eyes

Vitamin A is required to fill the night vision cells (rods) with a light-sensitive pigment called rhodopsin, and to produce iodopsins, the light-sensitive pigments for daylight (color) vision. Since vitamin A is stored in the liver, animal liver was the first "nutritional supplement" to be used to treat nutritional night blindness. It was employed for this purpose by Hippocrates who lived from 460 to 325 B.C. Cod liver oil, a natural source of vitamin A, was also found to remedy night blindness many centuries ago.

Vitamin A
A nutritional supplement required for the production of nighttime (rhodopsin) and daytime (iodopsin) pigments that are sensitive to light at the back of the eyes.

Researchers have identified only a small number of people (about 5 percent) with night blindness (retinitis pigmentosa-RP) who have a genetic defect that would respond to high-dose vitamin A.

The use of megadoses of vitamin A supplements for RP, or night blindness, is controversial. Some eye physicians recommend vitamin A supplements. Others do not, for good reasons. The problem is that, as vitamin A is used up in the night-vision (rod) cells, it is shed in small discs. These discs, as many as 25,000 per day, must then be digested by a layer of retinal cleansing cells called the retinal pigment epithelium, but these cellular debris cleaning cells are estimated to digest only 7,500 used-up discs of vitamin A daily. It is believed, therefore, that an accumulation of used-up vitamin A occurs in cases of night blindness, resulting in the formation of debris called lipofuscin. This debris blocks the pathway of nutrients into and out of the retina, which can cause the rod cells to slowly begin to die off. Giving more vitamin A would only worsen the problem, yet the prevailing advice is

to take high-doses of vitamin A for retinitis pigmentosa.

Researchers are experiment-
ing with ways to accelerate the
clearance of lipofuscin deposits from the back of the eyes by
sending a chemical signal for the
clean-up cells to digest more
lipofuscin. (See Chapter 3 for
phytic acid-IP$_6$ rice bran extract.)

Lipofuscin
*Used-up vitamin A
shed by the night
vision cells (rods) every
morning. Lipofuscin
deposits may cause
abnormalities in the
retina.*

Vitamin A Sources

Vitamin A is obtained solely from the diet, either
as vitamin A or as its precursor, beta-carotene,
which converts to vitamin A in the liver. Up to
a two-year supply of vitamin A is stored in the
liver. One international unit (IU) of vitamin A is
produced from 1.2 mcg (micrograms) of beta-carotene.

Sources of the fatty form of vitamin A (the liver
doesn't have to convert this into a vitamin) are
butter, liver, and whole milk. Sources of beta-carotene, the orange plant pigment that converts
to vitamin A, are apricots, cantaloupe, carrots,
chili peppers, dandelion root, kale, spinach, and
sweet potatoes.

Vitamin A Overdose

There is undue concern that excessive amounts
of vitamin A may be toxic in the liver. But a very
small number of people (less than 30 annually) develop this condition, mostly because of a
pre-existing liver disease. Vitamin A liver toxicity
may produce symptoms of brittle nails, dry skin,
fatigue, irritability, loss of appetite, loss of hair,
and nausea. Most cases of toxicity occur among
people taking more than 50,000 international
units (IU) of vitamin A daily for several years. While
high-dose vitamin A is believed to be potential-

ly toxic over the long term, there was a research study on a group of people with night blindness who took 15,000 IU of vitamin A palmitate daily for as long as twelve years and they experienced no symptoms or signs of liver toxicity at any point.

Vitamin A Toxicity

An abnormal but reversible buildup of vitamin A in the liver that alters liver enzymes.

A person would have to take a 100,000 IU daily dose of vitamin A for months before liver toxicity would occur, but, even then, the condition could be reversed simply by stopping the supplement. In 1980, the Food & Drug Administration conducted a survey and found that about 5 percent of all supplement users consumed 395 to 500 percent of the recommended daily allowance, with no symptoms of overdose reported. In the 130 years between 1850 and 1980, there were only 579 cases of vitamin A overdose reported, so over-dosing is not a common occurrence.

Overconsumption of beta-carotene cannot occur because the body converts it to vitamin A in a controlled manner. Excess beta-carotene is stored in the skin and may turn the palms and soles a yellow or orange color, which can be confused with jaundice. It's not jaundice if the whites of the eyes don't appear yellow, but sometimes this skin coloration is a sign of liver problems.

There has been one study that indicates that women who consume 15,000 IU of vitamin A from food or supplements experience a 3.5 times increased risk for having children with birth defects compared to women who supplement their diet with just 5,000 IU per day. For this reason, fertile females were advised to avoid food supplements that provide more than 10,000 IU per day.

Dosage for Supplements

The minimum recommended dosage of vitamin

A is 3000 IU daily for men and 2400 IU for women. An estimated 3 percent of Americans who take vitamin supplements consume more than 25,000 IU of vitamin A.

However, there is disagreement as to how much vitamin A is required for health. The National Cancer Institute and U.S. Department of Agriculture suggest 10,000 IU of vitamin A per day, of which 90 percent comes from plant foods as beta-carotene, or 5.2 to 6.0 mg of beta-carotene. On average, Americans consume only about 5,500 IU of vitamin A per day, which would mean supplementation should be widespread.

Vitamin A Deficiency

Hundreds of thousands of seemingly well-nourished American adults are deficient in vitamin A and may experience a diminished or delayed ability to adapt to low light conditions. Older adults or people with diabetes may have difficulty converting beta-carotene to vitamin A and they may benefit from foods or supplements that contain the already-formed vitamin A, as in liver and fish liver oil.

Among people with alcoholic liver disease (cirrhosis) or nonalcoholic liver disease, there is a severe decline in the conversion of beta-carotene to vitamin A. So the already-formed vitamin A is advised in cases of liver problems. (About 3,300 IU of vitamin A daily have been shown to successfully restore vision to alcoholics with impaired night vision.)

Poor absorption of beta-carotene or vitamin A may also result from celiac disease, Crohn's disease, pancreatic disorders, and other digestive tract conditions, which then can produce night blindness.

A very high intake of vitamin E can reduce the tissue and blood levels of vitamin A.

Zinc is also required for the proper metabolism of vitamin A, so a zinc deficiency may also result in night vision problems.

Vitamin B$_2$ (Riboflavin)

Riboflavin (vitamin B$_2$) is an essential B vitamin required for the production of an antioxidant enzyme called glutathione reductase.

Riboflavin (Vitamin B$_2$)

A light-sensitive essential vitamin. Too much or too little riboflavin can result in eye troubles.

A riboflavin deficiency may result in symptoms of burning and itching of the eyes, light sensitivity, and the growth of abnormal blood vessels across the cornea (corneal neovascularization).

A riboflavin deficiency may also result in cataracts. This would commonly occur among malnourished people, or those who have absorption problems due to a lack of stomach acid or digestive enzymes.

Excessive riboflavin may increase vulnerability of the eye structures to damage from unfiltered sunlight.

Riboflavin is also a light-sensitive vitamin. It turns brown when exposed to light so, when combined with exposure to unfiltered sunlight, excess riboflavin may induce brown cataracts.

Since our human eyes are transparent to light, excessive amounts of riboflavin may degrade our eye tissues. When rodents were placed on a high riboflavin diet and their eyes were exposed to ultraviolet rays, the light-receptor cells in the retina were shortened. The use of multivitamins is sometimes associated with the advancement of macular degeneration, and this may be due to excessive amounts of riboflavin.

When combined with sunlight, excessive riboflavin may promote the degradation of the vitreous gel that fills most of the eye. Excessive riboflavin plus unfiltered sunlight may cause the vitreous gel to liquefy or turn to water, similar to Jell-O that has become watery after prolonged storage.

Most vitamin supplements provide the minimum 1.6 mg of riboflavin, while some megadose vitamins may supply as much as 100 mg. Some nutritionists suggest 300 mg of riboflavin to remedy stubborn migraine attacks, but researchers have suggested that riboflavin be limited to no more than 10 mg from supplements. Vitamin E can counteract some of the adverse effects of excessive riboflavin in the eyes, but if you happen to be taking high-dose riboflavin under the direction of a physician, be sure to put on your sunglasses when outdoors in the midday sun.

Vitamin B$_3$ (Niacin)

Vitamin B$_3$ (niacin) is an essential vitamin in the family of B vitamins and is widely used in high doses to reduce cholesterol. Niacin in daily doses of up to 4,500 mg is often recommended by physicians, but this can result in retinal swelling, with accompanying dry eyes, loss of eyebrows and eyelashes (alopecia), loss of vision, and protruding eyelids (proptosis). All of these symptoms are reversible, so limiting niacin dosage to 1,500 mg per day eliminates them.

Vitamin B$_3$ (Niacin)
An essential B vitamin often used in high doses to reduce cholesterol.

Vitamin B$_{12}$

Vitamin B$_{12}$ is an essential B vitamin that is useful in disorders of the optic nerve and retina.

The importance of vitamin B$_{12}$ to vision is revealed in an experiment with monkeys. Caged monkeys were fed a plant food diet

Vitamin B$_{12}$
An essential B vitamin required to maintain the insulation (myelin sheath) surrounding the optic nerve.

exclusively, which provided little if any vitamin B_{12}, and were compared with a group of monkeys whose diet was supplemented with vitamin B_{12}. Even though none of the monkeys in either group developed signs of the pernicious anemia, which results from a vitamin-B_{12} deficiency, the group of monkeys that ate a plant-food-only diet exhibited abnormal lesions in retinal and optic nerve pathways. Although monkeys in the wild mostly consume fruits and vegetables, they do also eat small amounts of animal matter, which is a rich source of vitamin B_{12}. This study revealed that branches of the optic nerve (and probably other nerves throughout the body) degenerated due to mild shortages of vitamin B_{12} that did not result in anemia.

Heavy smokers may develop a condition called tobacco amblyopia, which damages the optic nerve and impairs vision. The nutritional antidote is vitamin B_{12}.

Vitamin B_{12} also protects against toxic reactions in the optic nerve caused by the release of glutamate.

In Japan, researchers used 1,500 mcg of vitamin B_{12} for five years on a group with various forms of glaucoma and reported improved vision or less narrowing of the visual field compared with a group that did not take vitamin B_{12}. The supplement protected the optic nerve but did not reduce fluid pressure in the eyes.

Vitamin B_{12} Counters Glutamate Toxicity

Glaucoma patients may lose some of their side vision without having elevated fluid pressure in their eyes. The pressure appears normal upon eye examination, but rather than there being pressure from the front of the eye, there are toxins slowly destroying the optic nerve. One of the nerve chemicals in the optic nerve is glutamate. As optic nerve cells die off from natural causes or toxins, they may release glutamate, which is toxic to the surrounding cells. Then, more and more cells begin to die off and release their glutamate, as happens in advanced cases of glaucoma. Vision that had been stable for years rapidly declines. In a laboratory dish, vitamins B_1, B_3, B_6, and B_{12} help to protect nerve cells from glutamate toxicity. S-adenosylmethionine (SAMe) has also been shown to be protective.

Glaucoma
Damage to the optic nerve from excessive fluid pressure, malnutrition, or toxins (tobacco, glutamate) that results in narrowed side vision.

The preferred form of supplemental B_{12} is methylcobalamin because of its absorption. In some studies, only methylcobalamin, not cyanocobalamin, the common form of B_{12} in food supplements, resolved optic nerve abnormalities. One study suggests that a daily minimum oral dose of 300 mcg of methylcobalamin would eliminate deficiencies in most people.

Folic Acid

Folic acid, a superstar vitamin in the family of B vitamins, is often overlooked for its role in ocular health. There have been few studies conducted solely on folic acid and eye disorders, but various wider studies have revealed that diets low in folic acid increase the risk of cataracts.

The likely link found between folic acid deficiency and eye diseases is homocysteine, an undesirable blood protein linked with Alzheimer's, blood vessel disease, and degeneration of tissues throughout the body. Researchers at the Medical College of Georgia have found that elevated levels of homocysteine, along with another nerve toxin called glutamate, can destroy nerve cells in the retina.

Americans are consuming about 270 mcg of folic acid from foods and supplements, and for-tification of foods has been boosted to reduce the risk of birth defects (spina bifida) in new-borns. But folic acid is easily destroyed by light and heat, so if foods like bread that are forti-fied with folic acid are heated, that can destroy much of this vitamin before it is consumed. Most multivitamins provide about 400 mcg of this vita-min. Recent studies indicate a minimum of 800 mcg of supplemental folic acid would facilitate reduced homocysteine levels. Betaine, vitamin B_6, and vitamin B_{12} also help to reduce homo-cysteine levels.

Vitamin C

Vitamin C plays a major role in eye disease. Since it was first discovered in the 1930s by Albert Svent-Gyorgi, a Romanian researcher, vitamin C has been known to prevent eye disease. Early on, researchers observed that retinal swelling and hemorrhages that occur in cases of advanced scurvy are resolved with vitamin C supplements. Just take a brief look at some of the research behind vitamin C for ocular health.

Researchers at the Human Nutrition Research Center on Aging at Tufts University determined in a recent review that adults with the highest circulating levels of vitamin C expe-rience nearly a 70 percent decrease in their risk for a certain type of cataract. An-other study shows a 77 to 83 percent reduction in the risk for cataracts when vitamin C

Vitamin C
An essential antioxidant vitamin that plays many roles in eye tissues, such as boosting glutathione levels, maintaining blood capillary strength, and promoting the production of collagen.

consumption exceeds 300 mg per day. Yet another study found that women taking 362 mg or more of vitamin C supplements experienced a 57 percent reduction in their risk for certain types of cataracts. So a 300 mg daily intake of vitamin C appears to be the minimum point at which cataract prevention occurs.

Another study shows there is little if any reduction in the risk of incurring a cataract among short-term users of vitamin supplements, but users of multivitamins, or any supplement providing vitamins C or E, reduce their risk for certain types of cataracts by about 40 percent. Cataract prevention has only been observed among those who took a vitamin C supplement for ten years or more, which is probably due to the slow progression of most cataracts. The positive effect cannot be observed until a decade or more of aging has passed.

It has been estimated that a delay of ten years in the onset of a cloudy cataract could cut the need for cataract surgery in half. Since more than a million cataract operations are performed in the United States annually, the widespread use of vitamin C supplements in amounts over 300 mg could eventually eliminate the need for cataract surgery in millions of adults.

A seldom reported study, conducted by researcher Allen Taylor with the U.S. Department of Agriculture Human Nutrition Research Center on Aging, at Tufts University in Boston, reveals that supplemental vitamin C significantly reduces the risk of both cataracts and macular degeneration. Of 300 women studied over a six-year period, 136 consumed a mean of 77 mg of vitamin C daily from foods and supplements, while 164 women consumed a mean of 294 mg of vitamin C per day. The risk for all forms of cataracts was reduced by 12 to 72 percent in these groups and the risk for macular degeneration was reduced by

52 percent among those who consumed nearly 300 mg of vitamin C daily.

In 1969, the Swedish eye physician Erik Linner reported that 500 mg of oral vitamin C, taken four times a day, reduced the fluid pressure in the human eye by about 2 points (mm/Hg). Interestingly, this fall in pressure did not take place until two days after taking the vitamin C.

Vitamin C is concentrated in the aqueous fluid of the eyes, which is just behind the cornea, the front window of the eyes. The aqueous fluid bathes the iris and the lens with vitamin C and serves as an antioxidant, or anti-rusting agent, to counter the undesirable production of free radicals as solar ultraviolet radiation enters the eyes.

The concentration of vitamin C in the retina is approximately twenty times greater than in the blood. High vitamin C intake has also been found to inhibit abnormal cellular debris, called drusen, at the back of the eyes.

Vitamin C Strengthens Capillaries

Vitamin C, along with bioflavonoids, strengthens the capillaries in the eyes that control the exchange of fluids, gases, and nutrients into tissues.

Bioflavonoids
Antioxidant plant pigments that bind iron and absorb solar ultraviolet radiation. Bioflavonoids work with vitamin C to strengthen blood capillaries.

When the blood capillaries are weak, the surrounding tissues will fill with fluid and swelling will result.

Hormones, such as estrogen, or stress hormones from the adrenal glands can weaken the capillaries and induce swelling, possibly even hemorrhaging. For example, during pregnancy when hormone levels are high, swelling may occur at the back of the eyes. In extreme emotional stress, swelling at the back of the eyes, a condition known as central serous retinopathy, can impair vision. It is, however, reported to occur more often in stressed middle-aged adults. Taking vitamin C, along with bioflavonoids, would strengthen the capillaries and produce an early resolution to these problems.

Vitamin C for Smoker's Eyes

It is not surprising to find that smokers have an increased risk for eye disease, including macular degeneration, which smokers develop about seven years sooner than nonsmokers. For every cigarette smoked, the body is depleted of about 25 mg of vitamin C. So a pack-a-day smoking habit would require the body to replace about 500 mg of vitamin C daily.

The amount of vitamin C in the body is normally about 2,000 to 3,000 mg, and the consumption of about 100 mg a day may maintain marginally adequate vitamin C levels. But physical or emotional stress, sunlight, medications, tobacco use, and disease may call for more vitamin C.

Americans typically consume about 110 mg of vitamin C from their diet, though the intake of vitamin C among those who do not eat fruits and vegetables may be less than 60 mg per day, which could produce marginal symptoms of scurvy. (Overt signs of scurvy don't occur until the amount of vitamin C in the body is reduced to about 300 mg.) Consumption of the recommended five to seven servings of fruits and vegetables daily would provide about 200 to 250 mg of vitamin C.

Take into consideration the fact that our bodies once produced their own vitamin C via the enzymatic conversion of circulating blood sugars as they passed through the liver. It is believed that we once produced anywhere from 2,000 to 13,000 mg of vitamin C per day via this enzymatic process. During periods of stress we would have produced more vitamin C, since stored sugars are dumped into the blood when there is physical or emotional stress. But somewhere back in our history, a mutation occurred and the gene to produce a critical enzyme for this process became dysfunctional so, from that point on, we have had to acquire our vitamin C totally from the diet. (Most animals, by the way, still produce their own vitamin C.) Judging by the amounts produced in our own bodies when they were capable of so doing, we can conclude that we should be supplementing our diet with at least 2,000 mg of vitamin C per day.

Bioflavonoids, pigments found in the rind of citrus fruit and in berries, cherries, and grapes, are companions to vitamin C that help to maintain the vitamin C levels in the blood. Bioflavonoids often accompany vitamin C in food supplements and should be at least 70 percent of the vitamin C dosage in order to strengthen the capillaries and prolong the action of vitamin C in the blood. In other words, 100 mg of vitamin C should be accompanied by 70 mg of bioflavonoids.

Vitamin E (Tocopherols, Tocotrienols)

Solar Ultraviolet Radiation
A spectrum of invisible sunlight that generates free radicals and may damage eye tissues.

Vitamin E is the anti-rusting agent for fatty tissues in our bodies and protects the fatty tissues from turning rancid. In our eyes, vitamin E is helpful in preventing cataracts and retinal disorders.

Vitamin E is required to protect the vulnerable light receptor cells at the back of the eyes, which are rich in unsaturated fats (omega-3s). Solar radiation can damage fatty tissues at the back of the eyes, but vitamin E steps in to prevent this from occurring.

Since the light receptor cells at the back of the eyes are insulated with unsaturated fats, vitamin E is required to maintain the proper function of these cells. Supplemental vitamin E may be helpful in preventing retinal detachment following surgery on the vitreous humor gel or the retina.

Retinal Pigment Epithelium
Also known as the retinal cleansing layer, this is a single-cell thick layer behind the light receptor cells in the retina that digest or clean up cellular debris and germs.

Antioxidant Enzyme

Vitamin E and the trace mineral selenium combine to produce an antioxidant enzyme at the back of the eyes called glutathione peroxidase. This enzyme helps to digest cellular debris in a retinal cell layer called the retinal pigment epithelium, also known as the retinal cleansing layer.

Cellular debris is generated from used-up segments of vitamin A that are shed from the night-vision rod cells every morning. This debris is digested by the retinal cleansing cells. With advancing age, the action of the retinal cleansing cells may lag behind the arrival of the used-up vitamin A, and tiny deposits called lipofuscin can begin to form. These deposits can, in turn, impair the transfer of nutrients and gases (oxygen) to the light receptor cells.

The death of photoreceptor cells in the retina has been directly related to the accumulation of lipofuscin in the retinal cleansing cells. As the lipofuscin accumulates, melanin, a brown pigment that protects the eyes, is displaced. Lipofuscin deposits may be an early sign of macular degeneration or Stargardt's disease (juvenile macular degeneration).

Vitamin E-deficient animals accumulate lipofuscin in their eyes at an accelerated rate. A five-year study using 500 units of vitamin E daily showed very small benefit to patients with macular degeneration, but the slow progression of the disease makes it difficult to analyze. In animals, a deficiency of vitamin E results in lipofuscin deposits within just twenty-one weeks.

While a complete lack of vitamin E may result in an accumulation of lipofuscin deposits in the retina, taking more vitamin E supplements alone, without other supplements, may not necessarily work to cleanse the retina of existing deposits, possibly because larger doses than we can consume would be required.

Vitamin E also appears to reduce the risk of cataracts. Various short-term studies have been conducted on this, but more long-term data is needed.

How Much Vitamin E?

The typical American diet provides about 10 international units (IU) of vitamin E. Most food supplements provide 400 IU or more vitamin E. Some studies reveal that our eyes benefit more from the dry form of vitamin E (tocopherol succinate) from natural sources (soy) than from the oily form (tocopherol acetate). Recent vitamin E studies are beginning to suggest that food supplements provide all the forms of vitamin E, the alpha, beta, delta, and gamma forms of tocopherol and tocotrienols.

One animal study showed that when quercetin, a bioflavonoid pigment naturally found in red onions and red apples, was added to vitamin E, the combination was more effective in protecting retinal cells from oxidation than the vitamin E alone was.

Vitamin K

Vitamin K is the blood-clotting vitamin. Many decades ago, Dr. Arthur R. Keeney reported on the successful use of vitamin K among people with macular degeneration where the onset of the disease was characterized by an abnormal pro-thrombin time and retinal bleeding.

While only 10 to 20 percent of those with retinal disease initially exhibit bleeding at the back of the eyes, for those who do have this form of the disease, vitamin K may be helpful. Dr. Keeney reported that some of his patients experienced improved vision following vitamin K therapy. Dark green leafy vegetables are a rich natural source of vitamin K.

Multivitamins

There are so many varieties of multivitamins on the market that it would be difficult to determine their ability to prevent eye maladies. But then again, there are a number of studies using multivitamins that cannot be overlooked.

Macular Degeneration *The loss of central vision that usually occurs with advancing age.*

The usual dietary intake of antioxidant vitamins and minerals alone does not appear to appreciably affect the risk of cataracts or macular degeneration, hence the interest in multivitamin supplements.

The Age-Related Eye Disease Study Research Group reported on the use of a multi-supplement formula that provided 500 mg of vitamin C, 400 IU of vitamin E, 15 mg of beta-carotene, 80 mg of zinc, and 2 mg of copper. Using this formula, there was a significantly reduced risk for advanced macular disease. Adults from ages fifty-five to eighty were studied for a six-year period. Visual acuity is measured by the ability to read increasingly smaller letters on an eye chart.

After five years, the probability that a person would experience a fifteen-letter drop in their visual acuity was 29 percent for people taking an inactive placebo tablet, 26 percent for those who took a multi-antioxidant formula, 25 percent for people taking zinc, and 23 percent for those who took zinc plus antioxidants. Really not much difference, but this study drew worldwide headlines.

There was a small increase in anemia among those who took zinc, and there was a yellowing of the skin among those who took antioxidants, probably due to the storage of beta-carotene in the skin. Interestingly, the mortality rate for the study group during this period of time was about half that of the general population! Not a word was said about this in the news reports.

Macula
Visual center of the retina that is primarily composed of color vision cells (cones).

The study did not indicate that food supplements prevented the onset of macular degeneration, nor that they improved vision among those who already had the disease. But it did prove that antioxidant supplements, if taken for the next five years by all six million Americans in the intermediate stage of macular degeneration, would keep about 250,000 of them from experiencing vision loss. In other words, antioxidants plus zinc inhibit the progression, but not the onset, of the disease.

Another large study, conducted among physicians in the United States, found that those doctors who used multivitamins of any kind experienced about a 25 percent decline in their need for cataract surgery.

Why Multivitamins Don't Always Work

One study conducted a decade ago showed that adults who did not take vitamin supplements had a lower risk for macular degeneration. This could be because few multivitamins provide an adequate amount of lutein and zeaxanthin, now found to be key nutrients to protect against macular degeneration. Most multivitamins provide beta-carotene and this competes with lutein for absorption in the diet. Taking the wrong kinds of food supplements has been associated with both early and late-stage macular degeneration, but it could also be because the studies are not conducted for a long enough period of time. Cataracts and macular degeneration progress slowly, and noticeable differences in vision and eye pathology are unlikely to be found in studies lasting less than a decade.

Lutein and Zeaxanthin
Yellow plant pigments that accumulate at the back of the eyes and act as internal sunglass filters.

The Beaver Dam eye study of 3,684 Wisconsin residents between forty-three and eighty-six years old found that adults who took multivitamins for five years, or took supplemental vitamins C or E for ten years, experienced a reduction in their risk for developing cataracts.

The severity of macular degeneration tends to be worse among those who have lower circulating levels of vitamin E and zinc and tend to be exposed to more solar UV radiation. However, an investigation known as the Blue Mountains Eye Study reviewed 2,873 people aged forty-nine to ninety-seven years and found no reduced risk for macular degeneration among users of vitamin and zinc supplements. So the studies can sometimes be confusing.

CHAPTER 2

MINERALS

Minerals are essential for our health, but because there is the potential for overload and side effects, mineral balance is very important, particularly between calcium and magnesium, potassium and sodium, and copper and zinc. Minerals such as copper, manganese, selenium, and zinc are cofactors in the production of antioxidant enzymes and may work in indirect ways to maintain ocular health. And magnesium is necessary for the enzymatic conversion of omega-3 fatty acids into DHA, a form of fat that insulates the retinal light receptor cells. Zinc is needed to mobilize vitamin A from the liver so it can be transported to the retina to produce melanin, a protective pigment in the eyes. An excess of minerals can produce undesirable side effects, such as calcifications in eye tissues. Copper and iron that has been jolted free from binding proteins by an overdose can generate free radicals that virtually rust away the surrounding tissues in the eyes. A lot of studies are being done on minerals, and researchers are gaining new understandings of how to control copper and iron to prevent eye disease.

Calcium and Magnesium

While calcium is a widely heralded mineral for bone health, magnesium deficiencies are far more widespread and are often unreported. Because of the interplay between calcium and magnesium in ocular health, they are discussed together below.

Magnesium plays at least four major roles in the health of the eye. First, it balances calcium by relaxing the smooth muscles that calcium constricts, and the interplay between these two minerals produces muscle tone. For example, a condition called blepharospasm, where the eyelids twitch uncontrollably, can often be remedied by simply taking magnesium supplements. Ocular migraines (pain behind or around the eyes) often occur when hormone (estrogen, stress hormones) or sugar levels are high, which results in a spasm of the arteries surrounding the eyes. Acting as a muscle relaxant, magnesium can help prevent ocular migraines by relaxing the spasms.

Arterial spasm in eye tissues can impair circulation there and damage the optic nerve. People with Raynaud's phenomenon, who experience poor circulation and numbness in their fingertips when placed in cold water, are prone to eye problems caused by arterial spasm. Again, a good natural antidote would be magnesium.

Second, magnesium helps to prevent harmful, excessive influx of calcium into cells. As such, magnesium is a natural calcium blocker, which can help prevent calcifications in tissues of the eye. Calcium is an essential mineral, but in ocular tissues it can accumulate in the focusing lens, which can, in turn, accelerate the onset of cloudy cataracts. Any calcifications in Bruch's membrane, a thin membrane at the back of the eyes, may impair the exchange of nutrients and the elimination of cellular debris (the exchange of fluids across Bruch's membrane is normally reduced by

Bruch's Membrane
A thin permeable membrane at the back of the eyes, between the blood supply (choroid) and the retinal cleansing cells.

half about every 9.5 years). This type of calcification is more common among those who have the fast-progressive, and more severe form of macular degeneration.

Third, magnesium protects the optic nerve and the other nervous tissues at the back of the eyes from overstimulation, or what is called excitotoxicity.

Fourth, magnesium (along with vitamin B$_6$) is required for the enzymatic conversion of omega-3 fatty acids in the liver into longer-chain molecules called DHA (docosahaenoic acid), which are transported to the retina and line the photoreceptors.

Low Magnesium Consumption

About 100 years ago, Americans consumed about 500 mg of magnesium in their daily diet. Today the intake of magnesium is only about 225–275 mg. Contrary to this, and largely due to the consumption of dairy products, Americans consume about 800 mg of calcium, which produces an intake ratio of about 2.5 to 1 in favor of calcium. This shortage of magnesium, which affects about eight in ten Americans, may be a primary factor in ocular disorders.

The ratio of calcium to magnesium in the human skeleton was found to be about two to one in favor of calcium. Nutritionists long ago recommended that twice as much calcium as magnesium should be consumed in the daily diet, though this was only a rough estimate of the proper ratio of these minerals. The two-to-one ratio of calcium over magnesium did not take into consideration the balance between calcium and magnesium required for muscle tone. We should probably consume a more equal one-to-one ratio of calcium and magnesium.

While magnesium is provided in foods such as green leafy vegetables and nuts, it is not likely that consumption of these foods would make up for the widespread shortage of this mineral in the American population, so magnesium supplements should probably be considered for everyone across the board. Taking magnesium supplements, 200–400 mg daily, would likely make up for most shortages. Too much magnesium could over-relax smooth muscles and produce loose stools, a problem that is easily overcome by reducing dosage.

Iron

A shortage of iron, or the release of unbound iron in ocular tissues, may spell trouble for the eyes.

Anemia, a shortage of oxygen-carrying red blood cells, is measured as a low hemoglobin level. The severe iron deficiency in anemia, more common in women than men, may cause a thinning of the whites of the eyes, the sclera. It becomes so thin that the underlying veins become visible and they give the sclera a blue tinge.

Iron-deficient anemia may result in a condition called papilledema, a swelling at the back of the eyes. This condition can cause cold hands and feet, a craving for ice or tomatoes, fatigue, pale skin, or symptoms of dizziness when you go from sitting or lying down to a stand-up position. Taking supplemental iron usually rectifies the condition.

Controlling Iron

While iron is required to produce hemoglobin, the oxygen-carrying pigment in red blood cells, it is also the body's primary rusting or oxidizing agent. It is important to understand how the body controls iron in order to know how to keep it from rusting out eye tissues.

In red blood cells, iron is bound to the red hemoglobin pigment. The liver also produces proteins, such as ferritin, lactoferrin, and transferrin, to bind iron so it cannot become a rusting agent. In the eye, such parts as the retina and the iris contain melanin, a brown pigment that helps to bind and control iron so it does not become an oxidizing agent. It is interesting to note that, as melanin levels at the back of the eyes begin to decline, the onset of macular degeneration (loss of central vision) is observed.

When iron is unbound, it can destroy living tissues by generating the most powerful rusting agent in the body, the hydroxyl radical.

Problems with handling iron become apparent in the eye when unbound iron is released in tissues, such as when hemorrhages occur at the back of the eyes. Small hemorrhages behind the retina, which commonly occur with advancing age, may release iron that can then degrade the vulnerable fatty insulation that surrounds retinal light receptor cells (rods and cones).

Mineral Deposits in the Focusing Lens

Chelation
The removal of metals by the attachment of ions to an amino acid (protein).

The focusing lens of the eye can accumulate minerals, such as iron, along with cadmium, calcium, and magnesium. The accumulation of these minerals may then cloud up the normally clear crystalline lens, inducing a cataract. Smoking tobacco increases the iron levels in the lens. Removal, or chelation, of these minerals may be therapeutic, reversing the clouding of the lens.

Minerals at the Back of the Eyes

Unbound iron and copper are the primary rusting agents that break down the vitreous jelly that fills most of the eye, which can then lead to vitreous and retinal detachment.

When iron is injected into the back of animal

eyes, there is accelerated accumulation of lipofuscin garbage deposits in the light receptor cells and the retinal cleansing cells, which results in deteriorating conditions in the eye.

Floaters
Clumps of protein in the clear vitreous jelly that fills the eyes and casts a shadow onto the retina, producing abnormal symptoms of cobwebs or blotches in the visual field.

Excessive iron levels in iron overload disease (hemochromatosis) can damage the tear glands, which can result in a chronic dry eye condition.

Mineral Chelators

The potential use of mineral removers (chelators) to treat ocular conditions in the retina and lens is overlooked. Desferal, an injectable drug that is an extremely strong metal chelator, may induce cataracts and abnormalities at the back of the eyes with just a single dose. So eye physicians shy away from its use.

There are, however, natural iron and metal chelators—the bioflavonoid pigments found in berries (such as bilberry, blueberry, and cranberry), cherries, citrus rind, grapes, and green tea; phytic acid (IP_6) obtained from rice bran; and quercetin (from red onions and apples). (See Chapter 7 for bioflavonoids and Chapter 3 for phytic acid—IP_6 rice-bran extract.)

Selenium

Selenium is an important trace mineral. It has been intensively studied in conjunction with vitamin E for its role in the retinal cleansing cells (retinal pigment epithelium) of the eye.

Selenium, along with vitamin E, is required to produce an antioxidant enzyme called glutathione peroxidase. This enzyme helps to clean up cellular debris as it accumulates at the back of the eyes. Selenium is 100 times more concentrated in the retinal cleansing cells than in the retina itself.

Macular degeneration is associated with lower levels of glutathione peroxidase in red blood cells, and people with macular degeneration have been found to have lower levels of selenium.

Glutathione
The master anti-oxidant produced in all living cells. Sulfur is required for the production of glutathione.

Supplementation with inorganic selenium (selenate, selenite), the most common form of selenium provided in food supplements, was not found to raise selenium levels among people with macular degeneration. Since selenium is readily absorbed from foods, organically bound selenium, the type found in plant foods, is the desirable form of supplemental selenium. Look for selenomethionine or SelenoExcel on the label.

Americans consume about 110 mcg of selenium from their diet, but there is a wide variance in consumption depending upon the selenium content in the soil, which varies in different parts of the country. Supplements usually provide 100–200 mcg of this trace mineral.

Zinc

The role of zinc in the our eyes is intriguing, particularly in our retinas where zinc supplements are now reported to be beneficial.

A zinc deficiency can result in alopecia, the loss of hair from the lashes and eyebrows, or it may result in cloudy cataracts. Zinc mobilizes vitamin A from the liver and works in tandem with it to facilitate night vision. In cases of night blindness induced by alcoholic liver disease, celiac sprue (where zinc is poorly absorbed), or pancreatitis, both zinc and vitamin A supplements may be helpful in restoring some vision. Since zinc is important for the conversion of vitamin A into rhodopsin, the light-sensitive pigment that produces vision in the rod (night vision) cells, supplemental zinc is often given with vitamin A. People with pancreatic inflammation who develop night vision problems should supplement with zinc, vitamin A, and pancreatic enzymes because this triple-supplement therapy has been shown to restore their night vision.

Zinc is needed by the melanosomes, the melanin-producing cells in the eyes. Melanin is required to control heat at the front of the eyes, to bind iron so it won't rust out ocular tissues, and to block oxidizing reactions caused by solar radiation. Pigs placed on a zinc-deficient diet produce an abnormal type of melanin.

Melanin
A brown pigment that binds to metals. It helps to control metals and heat in the eyes.

Zinc Controls Metals

All the tissues in the body, including the retina, must tightly control the metals in the body. One of the molecules that helps bind and control metals is called metallothionein. Metallothionein binds to cadmium, copper, mercury, and zinc as well as other heavy metals. Retinas with macular degeneration show a four-fold reduction in zinc levels, which, in turn, results in lower metallothionein levels. Zinc also produces catalase, an antioxidant enzyme in the retina. There is an age-related decline in both catalase and metallothionein in people with macular degeneration.

When placed in a laboratory dish with no zinc, retinal cleansing cells (retinal pigment epithelium) are very vulnerable to oxidation. Adding zinc to the lab dish protects these cells from damage.

Studies Are Compelling

Our retinas have the highest concentration of zinc of all the tissues in our eyes. In 1988, David A. Newsome and his colleagues were the first to report that high-dose zinc may prevent vision loss due to macular degeneration. The people in their study were given 100 mg of zinc sulfate twice a day. Over a five-year period, 78 percent of those taking zinc supplements maintained stable vision and 22 percent experienced very slight visual decline. Only one of the thirty-two people with macular degeneration who had taken zinc for five years developed macular degeneration in the second eye. For comparison, about one in ten older adults in the population at large experience loss of central vision due to macular degeneration. Men had less vision loss than women in this study. But another study that employed 200 mg of oral zinc sulfate had no effect on the course of macular degeneration over a two-year period. So it is uncertain whether high-dose supplemental zinc is beneficial for this disease.

Wet Macular Degeneration
Occurs in a small percentage of adults with this retinal disease. It is characterized by swelling, hemorrhage, or the development of abnormal blood vessels.

A more recent study that lasted ten years followed 66,572 women and 37,636 men who were over fifty years of age and had no previous diagnosis of macular degeneration. During that time, 384 cases of macular degeneration were diagnosed, 189 of which were the fast-progressing type of the disease (wet macular degeneration). Men and women who consumed the most zinc (25 to 40 mg per day from food or supplements) did not experience any lower risk for macular degeneration than others who consumed only 8.5 to 9.9 mg of zinc per day. So supplemental zinc is no magic-bullet remedy for macular disease, and increasing the dosage may or may not be beneficial.

Eye Doctors Change Their Minds

A recent study may have changed the minds of most skeptical eye doctors. A food supplement regimen that provided antioxidant vitamins, beta-carotene, copper, and zinc slowed the progression of the disease from one eye to the other. Although it did not reverse or prevent the macular degeneration, it was able to slow the progression of the disease.

People with macular degeneration have elevated levels of zinc in their blood serum, but the significance of this is debated. Does this mean the body is excreting more zinc or that it has a high zinc level? Read on.

How Much Zinc?

Our body contains about 2,000 mg of zinc, which makes it the second most abundant trace mineral. Zinc deficiency is fairly widespread, particularly among older adults. Zinc intake is about 10 mg from foods, but often only small amounts of this zinc are actually absorbed. Most food supplements provide about 15 mg of zinc, for a total intake of about 25 mg.

Zinc and copper must be consumed in the proper ratio to maintain healthy cholesterol levels—about a ten-to-one ratio of zinc over copper is recommended. Taking excessive amounts of zinc without any accompanying copper can raise cholesterol levels. Craig J. McClain and Mary A. Stuart of the University of Kentucky Medical Center, suggest limiting zinc to no more than 25 mg per day from supplemental sources.

The sudden removal of zinc from the back of the eyes is telling. Powerful zinc chelators, such as desferrioxamine, rapidly pull all the zinc from the back of the eyes, which can result in rapid loss of vision. Medications such as Ethambutol (a metal chelator) and Isoniazid may cause optic nerve problems due to the interruption of zinc absorption.

Copper

Copper is another essential metal in the body that must be tightly controlled otherwise it can generate rust and destroy tissues.

Arcus
A gray cholesterol ring on the inside of the cornea. This often occurs in later years and may be an indication of high cholesterol.

Copper is one of the metals that may harden (oxidize) cholesterol. Sometimes high cholesterol levels can become visually apparent as a gray ring of cholesterol deposited inside the clear cornea at the front of the eyes. This condition, called arcus, is seen in many adults of advanced age, but balancing copper with zinc may lead to the disappearance of this cholesterol ring. Zinc and copper must be in the proper ratio to each other for the proper handling of cholesterol.

Copper and Retinitis Pigmentosa (RP)

Some forms of retinitis pigmentosa (night blindness) are believed to be a result of chronic copper toxicity. Copper-chelating (removing) drugs like penicillamine have been proposed as a treatment for retinitis pigmentosa. In one study, all seven of the night-blind men and women who were placed on a low copper diet and who took a copper-removing drug experienced an improvement in visual acuity and a reduction of abnormal eye movements (nystagmus), and three of them experienced an expanded side vision. Zinc deficiencies are also known to result in diminished night vision, usually due to zinc's importance in vitamin-A metabolism. Another role for zinc in night blindness is its competition with copper for absorption. A shortage of zinc possibly opens a pathway for copper to become dominant in the retina, so balancing these two minerals is important.

Retinitis Pigmentosa (RP)
Night blindness caused by the disruption of the rod cells in the retina.

In night blindness, the blood plasma levels of zinc decline and the levels of copper rise. Chronic conditions, such as hepatitis and chronic infections, may cause a rise in copper levels in the blood. However, copper is only believed to play a role in the less common forms of retinitis pigmentosa. One study that used a copper-chelating drug with night-blind subjects who had accompanying hearing loss improved their deafness but not their vision.

Boron

Boron is a mineral known to help maintain healthy hormone levels (estrogen in females, testosterone in males). Through hormones, boron may indirectly play a role in ocular health.

Women who develop early menopause, or who have their ovaries surgically removed, are more likely to develop macular degeneration later in life. Women who are in menopause by the age of forty-five are four times more likely to develop macular degeneration. There may be two explanations for this. First, estrogen raises the level of good cholesterol called high-density lipoproteins (HDL). This good cholesterol transports a great deal of the lutein and zeaxanthin to the retina.

But if the HDL cholesterol levels are lowered because of reduced estrogen, this can impair the delivery of lutein and zeaxanthin to the back of the eyes. Supporting this viewpoint is evidence that the statin drugs known to reduce cholesterol also increase the risk for macular degeneration.

Hyaluronic Acid
The water-holding molecule of the body that provides support for all tissues and creates a barrier against the spread of disease. It is prominent in eye tissues.

Boron-Estrogen-Hyaluronic Acid

Estrogen is also important because it helps to maintain levels of hyaluronic acid throughout the body. This acid, a water-holding molecule, is found in high concentrations in eye tissues. Any breakdown and loss of hyaluronic acid can then cause a collapse of the support structure that surrounds the retinal light receptor cells.

While estrogen replacement therapy has been called into question in recent times because supplemental hormones do not reduce the risk of breast cancer or heart disease (though estrogen does reduce the hot flashes and other uncomfortable symptoms during the change of life), there is little question that estrogen supplements reduce the risk of cataracts. In fact, estrogen blockers such as Tamoxifen, a drug often prescribed to breast cancer patients, may increase the risk of cataracts by up to 400 percent.

Boron, by virtue of its ability to maintain proper hormone levels, may help to ward off the early onset of macular degeneration.

How Much Boron?

Dietary intake of boron ranges from 0.5–2.5 mg per day. The requirements for boron are not completely known, but a supplement regimen providing 3–10 mg would be safe and, as a bonus, boron has been shown to improve the hardness of bone and reduce the incidence of arthritis.

CHAPTER 3

THE MINERAL CHELATOR PHYTIC ACID

The human body accumulates metallic minerals (iron and copper) and heavy metals (lead, cadmium, silver, aluminum, mercury) with advancing age, which correlates with the increased incidence of eye disease in the later years of life. Calcium may accumulate as well, producing calcifications. Phytic acid, found in seeds and whole grains, is nature's mineral chelator (remover), and its application in treating eye disease is intriguing.

Phytic Acid (Inositol Hexaphosphate)

Phytic acid (IP_6) is a potent natural mineral chelator (remover) that shows promise for reinvigorating tissues in the eyes. Supplemental phytic acid may be helpful in several ways. It can remove calcifications from the back of the eyes (as in Bruch's membrane), which is an early stage of macular degeneration. It can remove the mineral deposits from the focusing lens of the eyes that can induce cloudy cataracts, and it can remove iron, a rusting agent that is released from red blood cells following a hemorrhage, from ocular tissues.

Also, because the progressive loss of melanin, an iron-binding pigment, signals the onset of macular degeneration, it is possible that phytic acid, an iron-binding nutrient, could make up for the loss of melanin in the retina by binding to iron.

How Does IP$_6$ Work?

Phytic acid is a component of whole grains and seeds. It is also known as IP$_6$ (inositol hexaphosphate) because its molecular structure is six molecules of phosphorus and one of inositol. Phytic acid works like a magnet to remove excess minerals from tissues. It attaches only to excess, unbound minerals and removes them via urinary excretion. Phytic acid has no affinity for the electrolyte minerals (magnesium, potassium, sodium) required for heart rhythm, so it does not interfere with them in any way.

Phytic Acid for Night Blindness

It is essential that the retina continually digest and remove cellular debris shed from the night vision cells (rod cells). This garbage-cleaning function is accomplished by the retinal cleansing cells, called the retinal pigment epithelium. They are really phagocytes, or digesting cells, and must digest thousands of discs of used-up vitamin A that are shed from the night-vision cells every twenty-four hours. When light first enters our eyes upon awakening, there is a burst of disc-shedding by these digestive cells, but if cellular debris accumulates faster than the cleansing cells can digest the debris, then some light receptor cells (rods and cones) are likely to die off.

The cellular signal for the retinal cleansing cells to clean up debris is sent by a molecule called inositol triphosphate, or inositol with three phosphorus molecules (IP$_3$). Carbachol, a drug commonly used to treat glaucoma, raises inositol triphosphate levels, and this has been shown to increase the ingestion of cellular debris from 9 to 34 percent. Vitamin D aids in the breakdown of IP$_6$ (inositol with six phosphorus molecules) to IP$_3$ (inositol with three phosphorus molecules).

The specific eye disease that phytic acid may

be most helpful for is retinitis pigmentosa (RP—night blindness), a condition caused by the failure of the retinal cleansing cells to clean up the debris shed by the night vision cells. Theoretically, taking supplements of phytic acid along with vitamin D, which aids its breakdown to IP_3, may be beneficial for people with night blindness. Although proven empirically over and over, there have never been any clinical studies done on this.

Dosage of IP_6

The American diet provides about 600–700 mg of phytic acid. The consumption of IP_6 from whole grains or bran from cereal will not remove enough minerals from tissues to be effective because most of the IP_6 is already attached to minerals. IP_6 as a food supplement is derived from rice bran and is processed so that 70 percent of the molecules are free to chelate. IP_6 rice-bran extract should be taken on an empty stomach with water only. About 2,000 mg would be a therapeutic dose accompanied by about 1,000 IU of vitamin D. An alternating regimen of mineral chelation using IP_6 with vitamin D should be employed for a period of no more than six weeks, followed by a six-week breather period. Continued use over a prolonged period of time can induce iron-deficient anemia, which may show up as cold hands and feet, fatigue, and paleness. IP_6 should not be consumed by pregnant women, growing children, or anyone who is already anemic.

CHAPTER 4

AMINO ACIDS

Amino acids are the basic building blocks of proteins. They may play important roles in ocular health.

Arginine

Arginine regulates a gas called nitric oxide, which helps to maintain retinal circulation at the back of the eyes. To demonstrate arginine's ability to widen the blood vessels in the eyes, the central retinal artery in animals was blocked for thirty minutes and then arginine was successfully used to dilate the vessels and restore circulation. L-arginine may also help to reduce abnormally high fluid pressure in the eyes.

Arginine-rich foods, such as chocolates, gelatin, and nuts, set up an environment that may trigger the eruption of the herpesvirus that is harbored in a majority of people. Avoiding arginine-rich foods is advised during any herpes infections of the eye.

L-arginine supplements are usually consumed in the range of 500–1,500 mg per day.

Carnitine

Carnitine is an essential amino acid that is widely consumed as a food supplement. With advancing age, or in a disease such as night blindness (retinitis pigmentosa), there may be an abnormal accumulation of cellular debris at the back of the eyes called lipofuscin.

Lipofuscin also accumulates in other aging nerve tissues, such as the brain. Acetyl-L-carnitine has been shown to reduce the accumulation of lipofuscin in the brain. However, although the use of supplemental acetyl-L-carnitine on children with a hereditary disease that promotes the accumulation of lipofuscin *did* remove these undesirable deposits from the brain, it did not remove them from the retina. Still, in adults, acetyl-L-carnitine may be useful following an ocular stroke (stoppage of blood supply) in the retina. Acetyl-L-carnitine is the preferred form of this amino acid in food supplements. Daily dosage ranges from 1,000–1,500 mg.

Proline

Along with lysine and vitamin C, proline is required to build collagen in human tissues. An age-related collapse in the collagen structure of the eyes would impair outflow of fluid from the front of the eyes (tearing), raise intraocular pressure, and subsequently damage the optic nerve. Among glaucoma patients, there is a measurable reduction in proline and taurine in the aqueous fluid of the eye.

The loss of collagen may also be involved in the elongation of the eye, a condition known as progressive myopia (nearsightedness). So proline is an important amino acid, and supplementing with it can be helpful in cases of common glaucoma and high myopia, though no studies have yet been reported using these amino acids for these conditions.

Taurine

Taurine is important to the retina and the lens. A sulfur-bearing type of amino acid, it is one of seven non-essential amino acids, which means the body can convert it from other amino acids.

Living cells are compartments of living matter made up of a fatty outer membrane that holds watery cytoplasm inside. Taurine is concentrated in these cell membranes to help maintain their integrity.

Cats Lack Taurine

Cats provide a good example of the importance of taurine in the eyes, since they can't convert other amino acids into taurine. Cats are almost totally dependent upon the diet for taurine, and a total deficiency induces blindness.

We have an even lower capacity to generate taurine than cats. In our eyes, taurine is concentrated in the retinal cleansing cells. The normal functioning of the retina requires taurine, and the combination of a taurine shortage with an exposure to potentially toxic radiant sunlight can induce retinal degeneration.

Taurine and Night Blindness

Does supplemental taurine improve vision? In one study, 1,000 mg of taurine and 800 IU of vitamin E administered to forty-four people with retinitis pigmentosa for up to forty months resulted in improved visual acuity (the ability to read two more lines on the eye chart). People with more serious forms of RP (X-linked RP) did not respond to this regimen.

A type of tranquilizer (chlorpromazine) and an anti-malaria drug (chloroquine), which are both light-sensitive drugs, markedly reduce the concentration of taurine, and both medications have negative visual side effects.

Taurine protects the lens of the eye from sugar cataracts, the kind developed in diabetes. Supplemental doses of taurine range from 500–1,500 mg daily, and zinc and vitamin E work with it synergistically to protect cell membranes.

CHAPTER 5

ESSENTIAL FATTY ACIDS

In the 1930s, researchers studied a group of Eskimos and found they were free of many chronic diseases, such as diabetes, glaucoma, heart disease, high blood pressure, and myopia (nearsightedness). These Eskimos consumed a large amount of cold-water fish that provided up to 14,000 mg of omega-3 and omega-6 oils per day.

Later, when researchers removed these unsaturated oils from the diets of animals, they did not thrive. From that point on, it has been known that these oils are essential for life.

During the intervening years, more processed foods have become staples of the American diet, and meat is fattened with grain at the feeding pen before processing, which reduces the available omega-3 oils. The result is a widespread deficiency of these essential oils, particularly the omega-3s.

A quick understanding of the nomenclature for oils is needed. Omega-3 oils are unsaturated and are derived primarily from fish and flaxseed. Omega-3s are the antifreeze for cold-water fish. Place fish oil in the freezer and you will notice the oil doesn't harden. So the omega-3s promote good circulation. Fish and flax oil also provide some omega-6 oils.

Omega-3 Oils
Oils derived from fish or flaxseed, which are essential for proper visual functioning.

The omega-6 oils, largely derived from corn, safflower, and sunflower oils, are also essential for health, also unsaturated, and they lower cholesterol. Corn, safflower, and sunflower oils do not provide any omega-3s. Omega-6 oils are dominant in the Western diet, to the exclusion of omega-3 oils. Omega-9 oils are the monosaturated oils and play no known role in the health of the eye.

Essential fatty acids, which are unsaturated fats, should not be confused with saturated fats, which largely come from animal products and are often involved in ocular and blood vessel disease. For example, studies indicate that the consumption of saturated fat raises the risk of macular degeneration, while unsaturated omega-3 fish fat reduces it. Adults who consume fish once a week are about half as likely to develop macular degeneration as adults who eat fish only once a month.

Fats Clog up the Backs of the Eyes

When animals are fed a diet that is high in poly-unsaturated fats, like corn oil, and their diet is intentionally made to be deficient in chromium, selenium, sulfur, and vitamin E, undesirable lipofuscin deposits form rapidly, within weeks. The deposits form in the brain, heart, intestines, and kidney, but more so in the eyes because they are bombarded by sunlight. Fortunately, these undesirable deposits can also be reversed. One study shows that dietary supplementation with a sulfur-bearing amino acid (methionine) and chromium reduces the amount of lipofuscin.

A high fat and cholesterol diet fed to small rodents results in the thickening of the normally permeable Bruch's membrane at the back of the eye, and this is believed to be an early step in the disease process for macular degeneration. The thickening of Bruch's membrane occurred within just fifteen weeks. As this membrane thickens, the transport of cellular debris, gases, and nutrients in and out of the retina is impaired.

There is about a ten-fold reduction in the permeability, or passage, of gases and fluids through Bruch's membrane from the first to the ninth decade of life. When the eyes of deceased people are examined, pathologists find a great variance in the thickening of Bruch's membrane among people of similar age, no doubt due to their nutritional supplemental intake over the years. As fats accumulate in Bruch's membrane, there is a decline in the number of blood capillaries that carry nutrients and oxygen to the inner retina.

Unsaturated fats may also harden or turn rancid in Bruch's membrane, which can inhibit oxygen transfer and excite the production of hormones that trigger the development of undesirable new blood vessels (a phenomenon called neovascularization). Since water and oil don't mix, the accumulation of oils and fats in Bruch's membrane may result in a hydrophobic state, that is, an impaired movement of water across the membrane. Fluid may then collect and force the nearby layer of retinal cleansing cells (retinal pigment epithelium) to detach. A pocket is formed and swelling occurs.

DHA Fat in the Photoreceptors

Omega-3 oils are converted into a longer molecule in the liver called docosahexaenoic acid, or DHA, a type of fat derived from omega-3 fats found in fish oil or converted from flaxseed oil, but an estimated 20 percent of Americans have no detectable levels of omega-3 fat at all in their tissues.

DHA is then transported to the retina and lines the retinal light receptor cells. Magnesium is required for the enzymatic conversion of omega-3 into DHA. This is of special interest since better than eight in ten Americans are deficient in both magnesium and omega-3 oils.

In the best of circumstances, retinal photoreceptor cells exhibit very high levels of DHA, The retina compensates for a deficiency of omega-3 fat by inserting omega-6 oils in its place. In animal studies, the provision of corn oil depletes the retina of essential omega-3 fatty acids, and this lack of omega-3 oils in the retina can pose a problem. For example, in the eyes of animals deprived of omega-3 fats, the levels of the night-vision chemical called rhodopsin are reduced, and there is a marked decline in their visual acuity.

DHA (Docosahexaenoic Acid)

A long-chain molecule derived from omega-3 oils that insulates the retinal light receptor cells.

Another example of the importance of omega-3 oils for our eyes can be demonstrated by the antagonism between alcohol and omega-3 oils. When cats were given alcohol to drink, the level of omega-3 fatty acids, which insulate the retinal light receptor cells, fell by 17 percent, and the ratio of omega-6 fats rose by 250 percent, enough to cause a loss of function in their nervous systems.

An Italian study using DHA-rich fish oil, vitamin E, and an array of B vitamins produced a beneficial drop in fluid pressure in the eye and an increase in peripheral vision.

DHA Increases Potential for Light Damage

While DHA is required for the proper functioning of the light receptor cells, DHA is also very vulnerable to turning rancid upon exposure to unfiltered sunlight, which reaches the back of the eyes. A destructive process called lipid peroxidation may occur. To prevent this, special anti-rusting agents, such as vitamin E, are required, In the case of retinitis pigmentosa, toxic byproducts produced from the degradation of DHA may gravitate towards the front of the eyes and cause a cloudiness on the back side of the focusing lens of the eye (a cataract), which can obscure vision.

Of all the cells in the body, the light receptor cells in the retina are the richest in DHA, and it appears to protect retinal cells during episodes of low oxygen supply. Patients with night blindness (retinitis pigmentosa) and Usher's syndrome have low levels of DHA.

The provision of DHA is very critical for the development of an infant's visual system. Infants fed mother's milk have better visual acuity than babies who are fed cow's milk. Mother's milk provides DHA to the baby's nervous system. Cow's milk does not. The need for DHA in prematurely born infants is even more acute. Infant formulas that provide DHA fat similar to mother's milk have just now become available.

About 3.3 to 3.9 percent of American adults over age sixty-five lose some central vision due to macular degeneration, and nearly a third of them have early retinal abnormalities such as drusen spots. In rural Italy, a study of 576 adults who largely consume fresh, unprocessed foods found only 1.1 percent of them had developed macular degeneration.

Moisturizing Oils

Oils from black currant seed, borage, and primrose provide an omega-6 type of oil that has been shown to hold moisture in the body. These are called the moisturizing oils.

Probably the most com-

Moisturizing Oils
Derived from black currant seed, borage, or evening primrose oils, these help to maintain moisture in ocular tissues as well as the tear film.

mon eye problem is dry eye, which produces the irritating symptoms of burning, itching, and redness. Eye drops provide only temporary relief for this condition.

Tear Film
A film composed of layers of mucin, water, and oils that coats the front surface of the eyes.

The most common reason for dry eye is a thinning of the oily layer in the tear film. The tear film that coats the surface of the eyes is composed of an inner layer of mucin (vitamin A), a watery middle layer, and an outer oily layer. The oils in the outer tear film help to prevent evaporation.

Dry eyes are often accompanied by other symptoms of dryness, such as brittle nails, dry hair, dry mouth, and dry skin.

Oils for Eyelid Glands

The oily tear layer is produced by glands in the eyelids. With every blink, some oil is squeezed out onto the surface of the eyes. Rapid blinking will deliver more oil and can help to temporarily relieve dry eye symptoms.

Dry Eye
A condition usually characterized by evaporation of tears from the surface of the eyes, or by insufficient mucin in the tear film, which produces symptoms of burning, itching, or redness.

A growing body of evidence reveals that, when taken orally, essential oils, particularly those from black currant seed, borage, or evening primrose, help to restore or maintain the oily layer of the tear film. Due to hormonal changes, dry eyes are a condition more commonly experienced by females over age forty.

Vitamin B_6, vitamin C, and zinc work synergistically with the essential oils from black currant, borage, or primrose. About 1,000–2,000 mg of these essential oils taken daily would remedy many cases of dry eyes.

Thickening the tear film with oral supplementation of essential oils will often increase ocular comfort when wearing contact lenses. These oils should never be applied directly to the eyes themselves.

CHAPTER 6

NON-VITAMIN NUTRIENTS

This is a category of nutrients that are not vitamins, minerals, herbs, or amino acids. These are called non-vitamin nutrients.

Coenzyme Q_{10}

Coenzyme Q_{10}, the nutrient for aging eyes, is an antioxidant produced naturally within the body. It is also available as a food supplement.

Coenzyme Q_{10} is important for the mitochondria, small bodies within living cells that produce cellular energy. Cell energy is produced by the synthesis of adenotriphosphate (ATP) within the mitochondria. Low coenzyme Q_{10} levels are an indication that cells are low in energy and cannot perform all their normal functions.

> **Coenzyme Q_{10}**
> An essential antioxidant produced naturally within the body that is required for cell energy.

For example, the cells on the inside of the clear front window of the eyes (the corneal endothelium) must be bathed with aqueous fluid from inside the eyes to receive nutrients since there is no direct access to the blood circulation. The endothelial cells have an inborn pump to maintain hydration, provide nutrients, and remove cellular debris. Cell energy is required for this pump action. Low cell energy levels may occur in cases of corneal edema (swelling), and taking oral coenzyme Q_{10} supplements would likely improve the pumping action of the cell. This may be especially important for anyone who has undergone a corneal transplant operation.

Most of the rusting, or oxidation, that occurs in the body happens within the mitochondria. There is a high energy and coenzyme Q_{10} requirement in the mitochondria of the retinal cleansing cell layer (retinal pigment epithelium) because these cells are so busy digesting cellular debris and killing off any invading germs. Coenzyme Q_{10} is potentially helpful in cases of retinal disease. A typical dosage of supplemental coenzyme Q_{10} ranges from 30–200 mg.

Mitochondria
Small bodies in living cells where the energy molecule (adenotriphosphate) is produced. This is where most of the oxidation (rusting) of the body's cells occurs.

Glutathione

Glutathione, the major detoxifying molecule in living tissues, is the king of the antioxidants in the eye. Glutathione is active in all the ocular tissues, in the focusing lens where it helps to prevent cataracts, in the fluid drain of the eyes to help prevent glaucoma, and in the retina to help prevent macular degeneration.

Glutathione is made in every living cell. Sulfur is required to produce glutathione. Glutathione is actually a triple molecule, three amino acids linked together—cysteine, glutamic acid, and glycine. Cysteine, the sulfur-bearing amino acid, is the primary nutritional factor that controls the internal production of glutathione.

As glutathione intercepts toxic free radicals and renders them harmless, it becomes oxidized, or used up, itself. Vitamin C donates an electron to glutathione and regenerates it, so making sure that vitamin C gets to the body's tissues will generate more glutathione than sulfur itself.

There are many sulfur compounds that can generate glutathione. Alpha-lipoic acid, cysteine,

MSM (methylsulfonylmethane), and taurine are all sulfur-bearing nutrients that boost glutathione levels.

Glutathione and Cataracts

Low glutathione levels are found in every form of cataracts (metabolic, radiation, sugar, sunlight, toxic, and traumatic). Even though glutathione was discovered in 1910 and was found to prevent radiation cataracts in the 1950s, slow progress has been made in glutathione research as an anti-cataract agent. Glutathione levels in the lens of the eyes decline with advancing age. The focusing lens of the eye loses about 1 percent of its transparency for every year of life. By middle age, glutathione is just barely adequate to maintain a clear lens, which is why cloudy cataracts occur in the majority of older adults, though only about 3 percent require cataract surgery at any given time.

People who chronically take acetaminophen, a common over-the-counter pain reliever, may experience a liver malfunction that will further reduce glutathione levels. For this type of acetaminophen-induced cataracts, glutathione is the antidote.

In animal studies, alpha-lipoic acid (sometimes called thioctic acid), which boosts glutathione levels, has been shown to reduce copper accumulation in the lens of the eyes and may delay the onset of sugar cataracts.

Glutathione eye drops have been employed in an attempt to prevent or reverse cataracts, with mixed results. Glutathione eye drops may not penetrate through the cornea.

Glutathione and the Retina

In the retina, most of the glutathione is found in the Muller cells, which reside in the nerve cell layer of the retina that carries visual signals to the optic nerve and then on to the brain. They are detoxifying cells that protect the nerve-relaying cells from damage by infection, inflammation, light, or toxins. In a laboratory dish, adding ginkgo biloba to Muller cells increases glutathione levels in the Muller cells.

A high level of glutathione is required for the normal function of the retina. Dr. Paul Sternberg, Jr., of Emory University, has demonstrated in a test tube study that retinal cleansing cells (retinal pigment epithelial cells) are protected from oxidation by glutathione.

Taurine, another sulfur-bearing amino acid, has been shown to protect the fatty lining that surrounds light receptor cells in the retina.

N-acetyl cysteine, another sulfur-bearing amino acid, has been shown to protect the retina from damage caused by intense ultraviolet radiation.

Glutathione and Glaucoma

Glutathione is the drain cleaner of the inner eye. It can cleanse the fluid drain of cellular debris that can abnormally raise inner-eye fluid pressure. High fluid pressure can damage the optic nerve and cause glaucoma. A small study conducted in Eastern Europe using 150 mg of lipoic acid, a sulfur-bearing nutrient that elevates glutathione levels, showed this therapy was beneficial to glaucoma patients.

Glutathione and Diabetes

Circulating blood levels of glutathione are lower in people with diabetes. After age sixty, more glutathione is used up or in an unusable state (oxidized) among those with diabetes and macular degeneration.

Boosting Glutathione

In tissues, glutathione levels may vary by sixteen-fold. The liver produces a back-up pool of glutathione to supply to ocular tissues as needed. The depletion of glutathione from the liver is associated with eye disease.

The consumption of glutathione from foods ranges from about 35–125 mg per day. Foods such as asparagus, grapefruit, and watermelon provide about 30 mg of glutathione per serving. However, the diet will not produce anywhere near as much glutathione as the liver, which generates as much as 13,000 mg of glutathione per day.

There is no recommended intake for sulfur, despite it being a critically important nutrient for human health. Sulfur-rich foods are asparagus, broccoli, Brussels sprouts, cauliflower, eggs, garlic, and onions.

Alpha-lipoic acid, a natural sulfur molecule produced within the body, is a unique antioxidant molecule because it is soluble in both water and fat, so it can penetrate to all tissues of the body. In animal studies, alpha-lipoic acid has been shown to prevent cataracts.

Typical dosage ranges for sulfur-bearing food supplements that boost glutathione levels are: alpha-lipoic acid, 100–400 mg; N-acetyl cysteine, 100–300 mg; MSM, 3,000–5,000 mg; and taurine, 500–1,500 mg.

Citicholine

Citicholine is a unique form of choline that has recently become available as a food supplement. It is able to penetrate the barriers of the retina and brain and is widely being studied for brain disorders such as stroke and Alzheimer's disease. Citicholine, when administered intravenously, has been shown to improve the electrical activity of glaucoma patients and, surprisingly, improved the visual acuity of patients with a condition known as lazy eye (amblyopia). The suggested oral dosage is 500–2,000 mg per day.

CAROTENOIDS

There is considerable interest in the role that colored dietary pigments called carotenoids play in ocular health. While there are about forty carotenoids in plant foods, about 60 percent of the carotenoid pigments in our bodies are only red, orange, or yellow.

Red (lycopene) is provided in foods like tomatoes and watermelons; orange (beta-carotene) is found in cantaloupe, carrots, pumpkins, squash, and sweet potatoes; and yellow (lutein and zeaxanthin) is hidden beneath the green chlorophyll in the leaves of kale and spinach.

Carotenoids
Red, orange, and yellow antioxidant plant pigments.

Beta-carotene

Beta-carotene's role in eye health has long been appreciated. The public is aware that Bugs Bunny's carrots are good for his eye health, and this is by virtue of their ability to provide beta-carotene, which converts to vitamin A, which, in turn, converts to rhodopsin and iodopsin, the light-sensitive pigments that produce daylight and night vision. (See Vitamin A in Chapter 1.)

Lutein and Zeaxanthin

The newcomer carotenoids on the block are lutein and its cousin zeaxanthin, which are being intensively studied for their role in retinal health and cataract prevention.

Lutein and zeaxanthin are concentrated in the very small central area of the macula called the fovea, which is only 1–3 millimeters across. Zeaxanthin is concentrated in the macula, but lutein is distributed throughout the entire retina.

These pigments are important for the transfer of oxygen to tissues, for protection from potentially hazardous ultraviolet and blue-violet sun rays, for sharpening vision by the elimination of unfocused light rays that enter the eyes, and for enhancing contrast and reducing glare.

Lutein is believed to convert to zeaxanthin in the retina. Also, whether the labels on food supplements indicate lutein is accompanied by zeaxanthin or not, all lutein-rich foods and supplements contain a small amount of zeaxanthin, usually about 10 percent of the amount of lutein.

Birds of prey are known to have very sharp vision, in part from the carotenoid pigments in the focusing lens and retinas of their eyes. Birds simply don't develop cataracts with advancing age as do humans.

Smoking and Carotenoids

One study showed that nurses who ate more spinach experienced a reduced risk for cataracts. It is interesting to note that dietary carotenoid consumption appears to reduce the risk of cataracts, but not among smokers. There is also a higher prevalence of macular degeneration among smokers, which may be partially explained by their having reduced levels of lutein/zeaxanthin. This is because tobacco interferes with the utilization of carotenoid plant pigments.

People who smoke need to eat more carotenoid-rich plant foods in order to retain good vision. A study of sixty-five people with macular degeneration and sixty-five healthy-eyed people did not reveal any differences in blood levels of beta-carotene, lutein, lycopene, vitamin A, and vitamin E. However, the smokers in the study did exhibit significantly lower levels of beta-carotene, lycopene, and lutein.

Yellow Spot over the Macula

When eye physicians peer into our eyes during an eye examination, they can often see a small yellow spot in the visual center (macula) of the retina. This yellow spot is the lutein and zeaxanthin that serves as a filter for the sun's rays as they approach the macula. Blue-eyed individuals have less protective lutein and zeaxanthin at the back of their eyes and are also at an increased risk for developing macular degeneration.

The macula is very small, less than two millimeters in diameter. It is where the color vision cells reside and it is what produces our central vision that we use for reading. Macular degeneration is a disorder of this portion of the eye that results in the loss of central vision, although the side vision remains intact. It is critically important that this portion of the retina be protected from solar radiation, especially from the toxic ultraviolet and blue-violet rays. Lutein and zeaxanthin are the sun filters for the macula.

In one study, the consumption of a 30 mg lutein supplement resulted in a 20–40 percent increase in retinal lutein and about a 40 percent reduction in the amount of blue light reaching the retina after just 140 days of supplementation.

Examining the Studies

The importance of lutein and zeaxanthin for the visual system was recognized as early as 1980. A two-decades old study showed that the removal of lutein and zeaxanthin from the diet of monkeys produced changes in the retina similar to those observed in human macular degeneration.

Up until recently, people with macular disease were told there was nothing that could be done for the common form of this disease. But everything changed when a 1994 report, published in the *Journal of the American Medical Association,* uncovered a relationship between diet and macular disease. Adults who consumed about 6 mg a day of lutein and zeaxanthin from plant foods exhibited a 43 percent reduced risk for macular degeneration. This amounts to about three to five servings of spinach per week.

Lutein Maintains Youthful Vision

A remarkable study conducted at the Schepens Eye Research Institute in Boston revealed that those adults who maintain adequate lutein and zeaxanthin levels in their retinas exhibit greater sensitivity to light. This is important because a gradual loss of light sensitivity precedes macular degeneration. But, with enough lutein and zeaxanthin in the retina, a sixty-year-old person was able to see faint light as well as a twenty-year-old!

Lutein Actually Improves Vision

In the most remarkable study yet, Stuart Richer, O.D., Ph.D., at the Veterans Hospital in North Chicago, reports that, in just twelve months, 10 mg of supplemental lutein measurably reversed certain aspects of macular degeneration, effecting such benefits as glare reduction, improvement in contrast, and the disappearance of blind spots. This is the first time that a food supplement has been successfully used to rapidly reverse this disabling eye disease, rather than just slow its progression or prevent its onset.

Researchers in Milan, Italy, reported an encouraging study where people who took a lutein/zeaxanthin supplement for eighteen months had their visual acuity improved by 25 percent, compared with an improvement of only 14 percent in a group that did not take the supplement. During the study period, vision worsened in 43 percent of those who took no supplements, compared with a smaller, 30-percent decline in vision among those who took lutein. This is one of the most encouraging studies to date.

Lutein for Night Blindness

People with night blindness (retinitis pigmentosa) who took 20–40 mg of lutein per day, combined with a regimen that included B vitamins, digestive enzymes, fish oil, and magnesium for twenty-six weeks or longer, experienced an improvement in their visual acuity, particularly the blue-eyed individuals. But another study, where lutein alone was taken, showed no improvement in visual acuity. So a combination of food supplements is strongly recommended.

Visual Acuity
The ability to read letters on a chart from twenty feet away.

Sharpening Vision

Lutein and zeaxanthin not only act like a sunlight filter for the retina, blocking out potentially harmful ultraviolet and blue-violet radiation, but also help to sharpen our vision by removing rays from entering the eyes that are poorly focused. Lutein and zeaxanthin also help to improve contrast, the ability to see objects in bright or dim light.

Invisible light rays, ranging from 280–400 nanometers, comprise the UV spectrum of light. Violet and blue light range from 400 to about 500 nanometers. Lutein and zeaxanthin filter out a significant portion of light rays, up to about 475 nanometers, or the majority of UV and blue light.

Lutein Reduces Cellular Debris

When retinal cleansing cells (retinal pigment epithelial cells) are placed in a laboratory dish along with lutein, zeaxanthin, lycopene, or vitamin E, fewer lipofuscin deposits are formed. These deposits in the retina are believed to be the first stage of macular disease.

Less Lutein in Disease-Prone Retinas

Macular degeneration begins in one eye and, over a period of about four years, develops in the opposing eye. Researchers recently examined the eyes of adults who already have macular degeneration in one eye and found that the other healthy eye contained less lutein and zeaxanthin than the eyes of adults who do not have the retinal disease.

The amount of lutein and zeaxanthin in the macula varies widely, by a factor of ten, with some people having virtually no detectable macular lutein and zeaxanthin. Women, who are more likely to develop macular degeneration than men, also exhibit less lutein and zeaxanthin in their retinas than men. Upon examination of donor eyes, investigators have found that the macular areas of the retina with the highest lutein/zeaxanthin levels are 82 percent less likely to experience macular disease.

There is a form of macular degeneration called Bull's eye maculopathy, which occurs when a person has been taking a photosensitizing medication, such as chloroquine. The damage to the macula looks like a donut ring, but the inner area of the macula is not damaged. This is probably because the yellow pigments, lutein and zeaxanthin, protect the central retina from sunlight damage and also help to retard the accumulation of lipofuscin in the central macula.

One study conducted in Germany found that lutein levels in the retina are reduced only in the late stage of age-related macular disease. Reduced lutein levels are not apparent in people who are in the early stages of the disease, or in the retinas of their offspring.

Relative Risk for Macular Degeneration Based upon Consumption of Lutein and Zeaxanthin

Daily lutein/zeaxanthin consumption	Relative risk reduction
1.7 mg	16 percent reduction
2.5 mg	23 percent reduction
5.8 mg	57 percent reduction

Dietary Provision of Lutein/Zeaxanthin

The intake of dietary lutein varies greatly in the population at large. Dietary consumption of lutein and zeaxanthin is about 1.75 mg in the United States. Zeaxanthin alone occurs about 170–187 mcg in the daily diet. (A microgram is $1/_{1,000}$ of a milligram.)

Every 10 percent increase in dietary lutein is associated with a 2.4 percent increase in blood serum concentration of the lutein. But only a very small amount of the dietary lutein and zeaxanthin consumed actually gets to the retina. Just 10 millionths of a milligram (10 nanograms) of lutein is actually deposited there.

Foods High in Lutein, per 100 Gram Serving

Amaranth leaves	15,000 mcg
Broccoli, raw	1,900 mcg
Cress leaf	12,500 mcg
Collard greens	16,300 mcg
Kale	21,900 mcg
Mustard greens	9,900 mcg
Okra, raw	6,800 mcg
Parsley, raw	10,200 mcg
Romaine lettuce	5,700 mcg

Spinach, raw   10,200 mcg

Foods High in Zeaxanthin, per 100 Gram Serving

Collard greens, cooked	266 mcg
Corn, sweet, canned	528 mcg
Kale, cooked	173 mcg
Pepper, orange, raw	1,608 mcg
Persimmons	488 mcg
Romaine lettuce, raw	187 mcg
Spinach, raw	331 mcg
Tangerine	142 mcg
Turnip greens, cooked	267 mcg

Lutein Transport and Storage

Some adults have virtually no detectable retinal levels of lutein and zeaxanthin. A study of twins revealed considerable differences in the lutein/ zeaxanthin levels in the macula, so there would not appear to be a genetic advantage.

The more lutein/zeaxanthin-rich plant foods consumed, the more of these protective pigments there are available for transport to the retina. Lutein and zeaxanthin require more dietary fat for absorption than beta-carotene. The consumption of dietary fat or essential oils improves the retinal levels of these protective pigments.

One study showed that there is an increase in the lutein/zeaxanthin levels in the blood of virtually everyone who takes lutein supplements. But only about half these people experience an increase in lutein/zeaxanthin in the macula after six months of supplementation. There may be an explanation or two for this connected with cholesterol.

Traveling on Cholesterol

First, all of the carotenoids are transported to tissues such as the eye on cholesterol particles, so any reduction of cholesterol may impair the delivery of protective and essential plant pigments to the retina. As women reach menopause, their estrogen levels drop, which results in a decrease in the high-density "good" cholesterol, which, in turn, increases the risk of macular degeneration. The association between menopause and the onset of macular degeneration could be explained by a decline in the delivery of lutein to the retina.

Second, since lutein and zeaxanthin are transported on fatty particles (cholesterol), they also can be stored in fatty tissues. Those who have more body fat are more likely to exhibit lower levels of lutein and zeaxanthin in their retinas, so greater body mass may limit the amount of lutein and zeaxanthin that gets to the retina. And, since lutein requires more fat than beta-carotene for optimal absorption, low-fat diets may also impair lutein absorption.

Cholesterol
Fatty particles produced in the liver that are required for the production of hormones and the transport of various fat-soluble nutrients (vitamin E, lutein, zeaxanthin) to the eyes.

Recommendations for Supplementation

Taking into consideration the dietary study that showed a significant decrease in the risk for macular degeneration among people who consumed at least 6 mg of lutein/zeaxanthin per day, and the fact that the diet provides only about 1.75 mg of these carotenoids per day, there is about a 4 mg shortage of lutein/zeaxanthin in the typical diet.

For this reason, supplementation is strongly advised for blue-eyed people, postmenopausal women, and smokers. The source of lutein/zeaxanthin in food supplements is marigold (calendula) flower petals. If the label on a food supplement bottle indicates it contains lutein, there is also a small amount of zeaxanthin included, regardless of whether this was noted on the label or not. More recently, zeaxanthin food supplements have also become available.

Lutein for Newborns

Newborn babies have no protective lutein or zeaxanthin at the back of their eyes and must acquire it from mother's milk. So it's a good idea for moms to make sure they are getting enough of these yellow pigments in their diet, recognizing that they now need to consume sufficient lutein and zeaxanthin for four eyes, not just two. Baby food (mixed vegetables, squash, spinach) is a reasonably good source of lutein for young children as they begin to be weaned from mother's milk.

CHAPTER 8

BIOFLAVONOIDS

Bioflavonoids, the antioxidant pigments found in citrus rind and the skin of berries, cherries, and grapes, are beginning to be better appreciated for their role in maintaining our health and preserving our visual system.

Bioflavonoids help to prevent cataracts; they reduce excessive inflow of fluid into the eyes and thus prevent glaucoma; they make up for the loss of the protective melanin pigment at the back of the eyes, which can lead to macular degeneration; and they strengthen blood capillaries at the back of the eyes, thus preventing the swelling and hemorrhage that often occurs when people with diabetes experience a rise in their blood sugar levels.

Bioflavonoids Work in Four Ways

1. Bioflavonoids exhibit antioxidant action by virtue of their ability to bind to rusting metals, such as copper and iron, and to the heavy metals, such as cadmium, lead, and mercury. Bioflavonoids bind to unbound iron, those iron ions that have shaken free from other binding molecules in ferritin, hemoglobin, and melanin.

2. Bioflavonoids work by prolonging the action of vitamin C in our eyes.

3. Bioflavonoids strengthen our capillaries and

help to prevent swelling and inflammation in ocular tissues.

4. Bioflavonoids also help to prevent overclotting of blood that can block circulation in the eyes.

It's amazing that the powerful properties of bioflavonoids continue to be overlooked in the treatment and prevention of ocular disease. A 1947 study conclusively showed that retinal hemorrhages emanate from weakened capillaries at the back of the eyes. Capillaries are the connectors between the red arteries and the blue veins. Taking 400 mg of rutin, a bioflavonoid derived from buckwheat, restored strength to the retinal capillaries and inhibited hemorrhaging.

A study conducted in France, where bioflavonoids are considered to be prescription drugs, found that a grapeseed extract supplement reduced the symptoms of glare that were produced when the eyes were exposed to bright light. Another eyebrow-raising study, which received widespread attention in the news media, revealed that moderate consumption of red wine is associated with a small decrease in the risk of developing macular degeneration. The bioflavonoid pigments in the red wine are believed to be responsible for this health benefit.

While a modern study dispelled the idea that bilberry (*Vaccinium myrtillus*) helps to improve night vision, this does not discredit the many other beneficial properties of the bioflavonoid bilberry for our visual system.

Bioflavonoids for Macular Degeneration

Bioflavonoids are helpful in preventing both common forms of macular degeneration. The dry form is characterized by the slow loss of central vision as photoreceptor cells die off or malfunction, and retinal cleansing cells (retinal pigment epithelial cells) disappear or become clogged with cellular debris.

The more advanced form of macular degeneration (called wet macular degeneration, neovascular macular degeneration, or disciform macular disease) is characterized by the development of undesirable new blood vessels at the back of the eyes that can invade the macula and obscure central vision, and by the pooling of red blood cells or blood serum, which pushes or detaches the retinal pigment epithelium from the blood supply layer (the choroid). Bioflavonoids help to maintain strong blood capillaries and inhibit the seepage of red blood cells or blood serum into spaces at the back of the eyes.

Stress-Induced Vision Loss

Physical or emotional stress may induce swelling at the back of the eyes and a sudden decline in vision. A condition called central serous retinopathy is produced when the capillaries at the back of the eyes are weakened, due either to the use of steroid drugs or to stress-induced adrenal hormones (cortisol), which can result in leakage of blood serum and subsequent swelling.

This is one of the most common conditions seen by retinal specialists, and it may also occur with people who have lupus, or when a woman is under severe stress during childbirth. One study found that a high proportion of people with stress-induced vision loss experienced a very disturbing psychological event just prior to their decline in vision. These people are usually middle aged (thirty to fifty years old) and in nine out of ten cases are high-strung men. This condition could certainly be called stress-induced temporary blindness. The vision usually normalizes without treatment, but there can be residual visual deficit in some cases. Supplemental bioflavon-oids, along with vitamin C, may help prevent stress-related eye problems. Certainly, as stress levels rise, it's a good idea to increase your intake of vitamin C and bioflavonoids.

Bioflavonoids that contain the dark-blue an-thocyanin pigments found in bilberries (Ameri-can huckleberries), blueberries, cranberries, and elderberries are the ones most studied in ocular disease.

Bilberry leaf does not provide any benefit to the eyes, so you want to look for bilberry fruit extract. And standardized extracts of bilberry are superior to non-standardized supplements. This means the bilberry is guaranteed to contain a certain percentage of the active bioflavonoid pigments. And Swedish blueberries are widely promoted and sold as a 25 percent extract.

CHAPTER 9

HERBS AND OTHER SUPPLEMENTS

Herbs were the first garden medicines for the eyes. Herbal products have been found to be beneficial for a variety of eye conditions.

St. John's Wort

Hypericin, the active ingredient in St. John's wort, an herb commonly used as an antidepressant, is a photosensitizing agent in the transparent human eye. Hypericin absorbs solar ultraviolet radiation, which means it can potentially damage the retina and focusing lens of the eyes. Appropriate precautions should include avoiding bright sunlight when taking this herbal remedy and wearing ultraviolet-blocking sun lenses because cataracts can develop upon exposure to unfiltered sunlight.

St. John's Wort
An herbal anti-depressant that may increase the eye's sensitivity to light.

Quercetin

Quercetin is found naturally in red onions and red apples. It is in the bioflavonoids class of iron-binding plant pigments, which makes it a powerful antioxidant. Oral quercetin is a natural antihistamine and is helpful in the treatment of eye allergies.

In high doses, quercetin has been shown to inhibit the development of sugar cataracts, as found in diabetes.

Quercetin also inhibits the herpesvirus and is

highly recommended if you have a herpes corneal infection. Also, it is a good idea to avoid arginine-rich foods, such as chocolates, gelatin, and nuts, during a herpes outbreak. L-lysine is frequently recommended for herpes infections, and it does help, but it is slow-acting.

Early studies indicated that very little quercetin is orally absorbed, but recent studies indicate it is not the quercetin itself but its metabolites, produced in the digestive tract, that are the active factors. As a food supplement, quercetin is consumed in doses ranging from 100–1,000 mg daily.

Ginkgo Biloba

Ginkgo biloba is an extract from the leaves of the ginkgo tree. It is a prescription drug in European countries but an over-the-counter remedy in the United States. It has been widely studied for its positive effects on circulatory problems, strokes in particular, memory loss, ringing in the ears, and other disorders. Ginkgo widens the small blood vessels in the brain, ears, and eyes, serves as an antioxidant (anti-rusting agent), and helps to inhibit blood clots.

In 1986, French researchers gave *Ginkgo biloba* to ten people with macular degeneration and compared them with others who received an inactive placebo tablet. A significant number of those given the ginkgo experienced an improvement in their visual acuity. Nine out of ten people taking 160 mg of *Ginkgo biloba* daily reported visual improvement, compared with only two out of ten who took the placebo tablet.

Ginkgo has been proposed as a therapy for glaucoma, but there have never been any clinical studies of this. There was one study, however, that showed that *Ginkgo biloba* was much more efficient as a retinal protector when it was accompanied by zinc.

The typical daily dosage of *Ginkgo biloba* is 120 mg twice a day, or 240 mg total per day.

Gamma Oryzanol

Gamma oryzanol is a nutrient found in rice bran that has been successfully used to control cholesterol. A study conducted in Japan showed that gamma oryzanol protects retinal cells from oxidation about four times better than vitamin E. Typical dosage in food supplements is 100–200 mg.

Coleus

Coleus forskohlii, a member of the mint family, is commonly used in marinating foods such as pickles. Coleus contains a compound called forskolin, which has been studied for its effectiveness in controlling asthma, cardiovascular disease, high blood pressure, skin problems, and weight loss. It is also widely known as a treatment for glaucoma. Because coleus herbal extracts may vary in potency, it is difficult to provide advice regarding dosage, so take according to label instructions.

Agaricus

Agaricus is a medicinal mushroom popular in Asian countries. Components of this mushroom help with wound healing and inhibit scar formation. Researchers suggest agaricus may be beneficial during wound healing following glaucoma surgery.

Soy Genistein

Genistein is one of the anti-growth factors found in soy. It works by inhibiting an enzyme called tyrosine kinase. When genistein is added to retinal cleansing cells (retinal pigment epithelial cells), it induces their death and renewal. Genistein may be therapeutic for the wet form of macular degeneration.

Vinpocetine

Vinpocetine has similar action to *Ginkgo biloba* but is not as well documented. Vinpocetine helps to improve blood flow. Dosage ranges from 10–30 mg per day.

Garlic

Allicin
The primary active ingredient in garlic that reduces cholesterol, kills germs, and controls blood pressure and blood sugar.

Allicin is the primary active ingredient in fresh-crushed garlic cloves. Topically applied allicin has been shown to lower fluid pressure in animal eyes under experimental conditions. But do not attempt to apply garlic juice to your eyes topically because the proper acid-alkaline balance may not be achieved, and you can damage the front of your eyes.

Although no studies have been conducted, it is possible that oral allicin supplements may be helpful in cases of glaucoma.

Ferulic Acid

Ferulic acid, an almost unknown antioxidant found naturally in bee propolis, blueberries, *Ginkgo biloba*, pine bark extract, rice bran and other plant foods, is an effective sunblocking agent against potentially harmful UV rays. Although ferulic acid has yet to be studied as a food supplement for ocular conditions, there is considerable interest in the health benefits of this natural antioxidant for nerve tissues similar to those found in the eyes, and for other sun-exposed tissues, such as the skin.

CHAPTER 10

HYALURONIC ACID

Hyaluronic acid (HA) is an important structural component of your eyes, and it is also concentrated in your skin and joints. HA plays an important role in the prevention of glaucoma, floaters, macular holes, and vitreous and retinal detachment.

Hyaluronic acid, the major water-holding molecule in human and animal tissues, is a very long alternating molecule of glucosamine and gluconic acid. HA binds salt and water so powerfully that just 1,000 mg of HA holds up to six liters (quarts) of water in living tissues. By virtue of its ability to hold water in a gel, HA provides structure to our eyes by filling the space between cells.

With advancing age, eyes actually shrink in their sockets, shriveling because of loss of water. Every decade, the eyes actually lose about 1 percent of their water content, and aging eyes also lead to a reduced amount of HA, a loss that is accelerated in diabetes.

A 1997 study shows that the clear aqueous fluid of the eyes of young children has a high concentration of HA, whereas in older adults it is almost six times less. Obviously the human eye is losing more HA with advancing age.

A report in the *Archives of Ophthalmology* measured the HA levels in the

Aqueous Fluid
The clear fluid in the front of the eyes; poor outflow of aqueous fluid may elevate fluid pressure and damage the optic nerve at the back of the eyes.

eyes. When eye tissues from adults who were over fifty years old and had failing eyes were examined, there was a complete absence of HA in tissues at the back of their eyes.

There is a matrix of connective tissue that surrounds and supports the light receptor cells in the retina. With advancing age, the loss of HA in this connective tissue may result in the inability to support the retinal cells, which can lead to folds in the retina, a condition called macular pucker.

HA and Glaucoma

The common form of glaucoma has been defined as a hyaluronic acid deficiency disease. The fluid drain becomes mushy and collapses with advancing age, which can cause the fluid in the inner eye to become trapped as it is filtered through the eyes, resulting in glaucoma. Cells obtained from the eyes of glaucoma patients produce less HA than healthy cells, and eyes with glaucoma exhibit an 80 to 90 percent decrease in HA.

In 1997, researchers at Boston University School of Medicine examined the eyes of people with glaucoma and found no hyaluronic acid around certain nerve bundles at the back of their eyes. Decreased HA in the eyes is symptomatic of optic nerve degeneration and of a high susceptibility to the elevated pressure inside the eyes that causes glaucoma.

HA and the Vitreous Jelly

Vitreous jelly fills most of the eyes and hyaluronic acid makes up 92 percent of the collagens in this vitreous jelly. As HA breaks down, it can cause water to be released from the vitreous gel, like Jell-O that has liquefied after prolonged storage. The eye then becomes mushy and loses its scaffolding structure.

The vitreous jelly may subsequently shrink and

detach from the retina. This unwelcome event commonly occurs in the fifth or sixth decade of life and typically produces symptoms of light flashes and floaters (dark cobwebs or globs in the visual field). HA levels are higher in eyes where the vitreous jelly is still intact. Once the vitreous is no longer filling and supporting the eye from the inside, the retina may also detach, an event that requires immediate medical care in order for vision to be preserved.

Lifelong bombardment by solar radiation, excessive riboflavin (vitamin B_2), the use of photosensitizing drugs, or the release of unbound copper or iron accelerates the production of hyaluronidase, an enzyme that breaks down HA. In one study, when hyaluronidase was injected into animals, it caused the vitreous detachment from the retina discussed above.

European researchers have shown that the temperature inside the human eye may rise upon exposure to sunlight, which also produces a breakdown of the HA. For this reason, it is a good idea to use sunglasses with mirrored lenses that filter out the heat-producing infrared rays.

HA and the Retina

Researchers have also shown that the wall of the eyes becomes more rigid and less flexible among people who have macular degeneration.

At the very center of the retina, there is a concentration of color-vision cells called the macula. This visual center of the eye is used for reading and central vision, and sometimes, chiefly among women, a hole occurs in the macula. A report in the *American Journal of Ophthalmology* links these macular holes with low estrogen levels. Since estrogen raises the levels of hyaluronic acid, it is possible that reduced levels of HA may give rise to macular holes, but it is not known whether or not supplemental HA would repair these macular holes.

Maintaining HA

Nutritional factors, herbs, and bioflavonoids, such as echinacea, grapeseed extract, IP_6 rice bran extract, and quercetin, help to stabilize HA and prevent its breakdown. Chondroitin sulfate, available as a food supplement, also raises HA levels.

With the onset of menopause and declining estrogen levels, women experience more eye disease. This is not surprising since estrogen helps to maintain high hyaluronic acid levels. For strategies to maintain estrogen and HA levels with advancing age, see the section on boron in Chapter 2.

Supplemental HA

Injectable hyaluronic acid is utilized in almost all ocular surgery to maintain the shape of the eye during the operation. Highly absorbable oral HA supplements have recently become available and they are restoring HA levels to the joints and the skin. Some of the people taking HA supplements reported that their floaters disappeared and they became less dependent on eyeglasses, but no controlled studies have been performed to date. Supplemental HA in the range of 100–150 mg per day is recommended.

CONCLUSION

The two eyes we are born with must last a life-time, and to maintain independent living, this vital visual organ must remain healthy. What we have learned in this book is that something *can* be done to stave off the inevitable.

Compelling studies point to the potential prevention of up to 80 percent of cataracts. Even if cataracts could only be delayed for ten years or so, the rate of cataract surgery would be cut in half.

Blind spots and visual distortions from macular degeneration have now been documented to clear up with nutritional therapy. It's not only possible to slow the progression of macular degeneration, but it's also possible to actually reverse certain aspects of this once-incurable eye disorder.

Glaucoma has remained a puzzling eye disorder because, even with very tight medical control of fluid pressure in the eyes, the side vision can be lost over time. The optic nerve must be protected from internal toxins (homocysteine, glutamate), and various antioxidants, minerals, and herbs have been shown to provide this protection.

The aging of tissues in the eyes progresses at a very slow rate. So the benefits of taking food supplements to prevent age-related eye disorders may not become apparent for some time. Various studies are now showing that lifelong users of food supplements begin to exhibit healthier eyes and better vision, compared to those who do not use food supplements. Now is the time to begin using nutritional supplements to preserve your visual capacity.

The human eye is an unusual organ. It is transparent to light, and is therefore vulnerable to bombardment by solar ultraviolet and blue-violet radiation. Lifelong exposure to unfiltered sun rays increases the risk of eye disease. So, in addition to good nutrition, UV blue-blocking sun lenses are strongly advised if you go outdoors in the midday sun. The habitual use of tinted sunglasses is especially important for blue-eyed people who have less protective pigment than people with darker eyes.

Eye Disorders and Important Nutritional Supplements

Cataracts   alpha-lipoic acid, glutathione, lutein/zeaxanthin, N-acetyl cysteine, quercetin, vitamin C

Diabetic eye disease   alpha-lipoic acid, bilberry, glutathione, quercetin, vitamin C

Dry eyes   borage, evening primrose or black currant seed oils, vitamin B_6

Floaters   hyaluronic acid

Glaucoma   alpha-lipoic acid, hyaluronic acid, vitamin B_{12}, vitamin C

Macular degeneration   alpha-lipoic acid, bioflavonoids, boron, glutathione, lutein/zeaxanthin, selenium, zinc

Night blindness   DHA omega-3 fish oil, IP$_6$ rice bran extract, lutein/zeaxanthin, taurine, vitamin A

SELECTED REFERENCES

Age-Related Eye Disease Study Research Group. A randomized, placebo-controlled, clinical trial of high-dose supplementation with vitamins C and E, beta-carotene, and zinc for age-related macular degeneration and vision loss. *Archives of Ophthalmology*, 2001; 119:1417–36.

Bone, RA, Landrum, JT, Mayne, ST, et al. Macular pigment in donor eyes with and without AMD: a case-control study. *Investigative Ophthalmology*, 2001; 42:235–40.

Dagnelle, G, Zorge, IS, McDonald, TM. Lutein improves visual function in some patients with retinal degeneration: a pilot study via the internet. *Optometry*, 2000; 71:147–64.

Gahlot, DK. Penicillamine: a new therapy of retinitis pigmentosa. *Indian Journal of Ophthalmology*, 1981; 29:355–58

Hammond, BR, Wooten, BR, Curran-Celentano, J. Carotenoids in the retina and lens: possible acute and chronic effects on human visual performance. *Archives of Biochemistry & Biophysics*, 2001; 385: 41–46.

Hammond, BR, Wooten, BR, Snodderly, DM. Preservation of visual sensitivity of older subjects: association with macular pigment density. *Investigative Ophthalmology*, 1998; 39:397–406.

Handelman, GJ, Dratz, EA, Reay, CC, et al. Carotenoids in the human macula and whole retina. *Investigative Ophthalmology*, 1988; 29:850–55.

Hind, VM. Degeneration in the peripheral visual pathway of vitamin B_{12}-deficient monkeys. Transactions Ophthalmological Society UK, 1970; 90:839–46.

Ito, T, Nakano, M, Yamamoto, Y, et al. Hemoglobin-induced lipid peroxidation in the retina: a possible mechanisms for macular degeneration. *Archives of Biochemistry & Biophysics*, 1995; 316:864–72.

Katz, ML, Stone, WL, Dratz, EA. Fluorescent pigment accumulation in retinal pigment epithelium of antioxidant-deficient rats. *Investigative Ophthalmology*, 1978; 17:1048–58.

Katz, ML, Norberg, M, Stientjes, HJ. Reduced phagosomal content of the retinal pigment epithelium in response to retinoid deprivation. *Investigative Ophthalmology*, 1992; 33:2612–18.

Knepper, PA, Goossens, W, Hvizd, M, et al. Glycosaminoglycans of the human trabecular meshwork in primary open-angle glaucoma. *Investigative Ophthalmology*, 1996; 37:1360–67.

Landrum, JT, Bone, RA, Joa, H, et al. A one-year study of the macular pigment: the effect of 140 days of a lutein supplement. *Experimental Eye Research*, 1997; 65:57–62.

Lebuisson, DA, Leroy, L, Rigal, G. Treatment of senile macular degeneration with *Ginkgo biloba* extract. *Presse Medicale*, 1986; 15:1556–58.

Malinow, MR, Burns, LF, Peterson, LH, et al. Diet-related macular anomalies in monkeys. *Investigative Ophthalmology*, 1968; 19:857–63.

Mares-Perlman, JA, Lyle, BJ, Klein, R, et al. Vitamin supplement use and incident cataracts in a population-based study. *Archives of Ophthalmology*, 2000; 118:1556–63.

Massacesi, AL, Faletra, R, Gerosa, F, et al. The effect of oral supplementation of macular carotenoids (lutein and zeaxanthin) on the prevention of age-related macular degeneration: an 18 months follow-up study, Program No. 1261, 2001. ARVO (Association for Research in Vision and Ophthalmology) annual meeting. Fort Lauderdale, Florida, USA. April 29–May 4, 2001. Abstracts. *Investigative Ophthalmology Visual Sciences*, 2001; 42:S1–945.

McCarty, MF. Primary open-angle glaucoma may be a hyaluronic acid deficiency disease: potential for glucosamine in prevention and therapy. *Medical Hypotheses*, 1998; 51:483–84.

McClain, CJ, Stuart, MA. Zinc metabolism in the elderly. *Geriatric Nutrition*, John E. Morley, ed. New York, NY: Raven Press, 1990, 161–68.

Newsome, DA, Swartz, M, Leone, NC, et al. Oral zinc in macular degeneration. *Archives of Ophthalmology*, 1988; 106:192–98.

Nicolas, MG, Keiko, F, Murayama, K, et al. Studies in the mechanisms of early onset macular degeneration in cynomolgus monkeys. II Suppression of metallothionein synthesis in the retina in oxidative stress. *Experimental Eye Research*, 1996; 62:399–408.

Obin, M, Nowell, T, Taylor, A. A comparison of ubiquitin-dependent proteolysis of red outer segment protein in reticulocyte lysate and a retinal pigment epithelial cell line. *Current Eye Research*, 1995; 14: 751–60.

Richer, S. Part II: ARMD- Pilot (case studies) environmental intervention studies, *Journal American Medical Association*, 1999; 70:24–36.

Robison, WG, Kuwabara, T, Bieri, JG. The roles of vitamin E and unsaturated fatty acids in the visual process. *Retina*, 1982; 2:263–81.

Robison WG, Kuwabara T, Bieri, JG. Deficiencies of vitamins E and A in the rat. Retinal damage and lipofuscin accumulation. *Investigative Ophthalmology*, 1980; 19:1030–37.

Sakai, T, Murata, M, Amemiya, T. Effect of long-term treatment of glaucoma with vitamin B_{12}. *Glaucoma,* 1992; 14:167–70.

Schweitzer, D, Guenther, S, Scibor, M, et al. Spectrometic investigations in ocular hypertension and early stages of primary open angle glaucoma and of low tension glaucoma, multisubstance analysis. *International Ophthalmology,* 1992; 16:251–57.

Seddon, JM, Ajani, UA, Sperduto, RD, et al. Dietary carotenoids, vitamin A, C, and E, and advanced age-related macular degeneration. *Journal American Medical Association,* 1994; 272:1413–20.

Smith, W, Mitchell, P, Leeder, SR. Dietary fat and fish intake and age-related maculopathy. *Archives of Ophthalmology,* 2000; 118:401–04.

Taylor, A. Cataract and macular degeneration: relationship to long-term ascorbate intake. *Clinical Chemistry,* 1993; 39:1305.

Weiter, JJ, Delori, F, Dorey, CK. Central sparing in annular macular degeneration. *American Journal of Ophthalmology,* 1988; 106:286–92.

OTHER BOOKS AND RESOURCES

Rose, Marc R., Rose, Michael R. *Save Your Sight!: Natural Ways to Prevent and Reverse Macular Degeneration.* New York, NY: Warner Books, 1998.

GreatLife Magazine
Consumer magazine with articles on vitamins, minerals, herbs, and foods.

Available for free at many health and natural food stores.

Let's Live Magazine
Consumer magazine with emphasis on the health benefits of vitamins, minerals, and herbs.

Customer service:
1-800-676-4333
P.O. Box 74908
Los Angeles, CA 90004

Subscriptions: 12 issues per year, $19.95 in the U.S.; $31.95 outside the U.S.

Physical Magazine
Magazine oriented to body builders and other serious athletes.

Customer service:
1-800-676-4333
P.O. Box 74908
Los Angeles, CA 90004

Subscriptions: 12 issues per year, $19.95 in the U.S.; $31.95 outside the U.S.

The Nutrition Reporter™ newsletter
Monthly newsletter that summarizes recent medical research on vitamins, minerals, and herbs.

Customer service:

P.O. Box 30246

Tucson, AZ 85751-0246

e-mail: jack@thenutritionreporter.com

www.nutritionreporter.com

Subscriptions: $26 per year (12 issues) in the U.S.; $32 U.S. or $48 CNC for Canada; $38 for other countries.

Websites

Lutein Information Bureau

www.luteininfo.com

The Lutein Information Bureau encourages you to look at lutein and its role in vision and overall health.

Author's Website

www.askbillsardi.com

Health journalist Bill Sardi will answer your personal questions regarding ocular health, as well as nutritional supplement regimens.

INDEX

Printed in the USA
CPSIA information can be obtained
at www.ICGtesting.com
JSHW012007140824
68134JS00004B/56